ACE VOICES

by the same author

They/Them/Their
A Guide to Nonbinary and Genderqueer Identities
Eris Young
ISBN 978 1 78592 483 5
eISBN 978 1 78450 872 2

of related interest

How to be Ace
A Memoir of Growing Up Asexual
Rebecca Burgess
ISBN 978 1 78775 215 3
eISBN 978 1 78775 216 0

How to Understand Your Sexuality
A Practical Guide for Exploring Who You Are
Meg-John Barker and Alex Iantaffi
ISBN 978 1 78775 618 2
eISBN 978 1 78775 619 9

Sounds Fake But Okay
An Asexual Perspective on Love, Relationships, Sex, and Pretty Much Anything Else
Sarah Costello and Kayla Kaszyca
ISBN 978 1 83997 001 6
eISBN 978 1 83997 002 3

I Am Ace
Advice on Living Your Best Asexual Life
Cody Daigle-Orians
ISBN 978 1 83997 262 1
eISBN 978 1 83997 263 8

Ace Voices

What It Means to Be Asexual, Aromantic, Demi or Grey-Ace

Eris Young

Jessica Kingsley Publishers
London and Philadelphia

First published in Great Britain in 2023 by Jessica Kingsley Publishers
An imprint of Hodder & Stoughton Ltd
An Hachette UK Company

1

A CIP catalogue record for this title is available from the British Library and the Library of Congress

ISBN 978 1 78775 698 4
eISBN 978 1 78775 699 1

Printed and bound in the United States by Integrated Books International

Jessica Kingsley Publishers
Carmelite House
50 Victoria Embankment
London EC4Y 0DZ

www.jkp.com

To us.

Acknowledgements

One hundred thousand thank yous to all of the people who shared their experiences with me: AK, AQ, BC, BH, CF, DC, EH, EL, EP, HBJ, HD, HG, JH, JTS, LG, LH, LL, LM, LV, NT, RH, RK, RR, SKW, SS, VC, and to those who remained anonymous, for your openness and generosity. Also to all my a-spec friends, especially CW, DL and SG: thank you for being part of my life. Thank you to Dalry Dinners, for putting up with my constant moaning. Thank you to Angela Chen, Lee from *Acing History* and all the others doing this work alongside me. Thank you to Mom and Dad, for never pressuring me to settle down and get married. Finally, thank you to Kez, for long chats about this stuff even when we're both tired, and to Annita, I'm glad we found each other when we did.

Contents

A Note to My Readers

Throughout these pages, you will find mention of topics that some readers may find distressing, including sexual assault, childhood sexual abuse, genocide, the transatlantic slave trade, forced sterilisation and corrective rape. I mention these subjects only in my exploration of the ways that a-spec people are and have been marginalised and do not go into detail, but I will flag them up at the beginning of a chapter, nonetheless.

A note on anonymity

The people who I spoke to in depth for this project, and whom I quote in the following text, were given the option to be either referred to by their initials or be completely anonymous. For those who chose to remain completely anonymous I have assigned a random combination of letters (i.e. "OC", "QL", "AZ", etc.) with no connection to their actual initials.

Introduction

I almost didn't write this book. There was a moment, before I signed the contract, when I seriously questioned whether I should be the one to take on a project that was – to my mind at least – so very important. I knew I was asexual; that hadn't been in doubt since high school, but I felt like I should confess to my publishers – to my *readers*, even – that I was not entirely comfortable with this fact. I hadn't yet (in the language I used back then) "come to terms with it": I didn't yet know how I could be ace and still have a future. Surely, I thought, the person writing this book shouldn't still be carrying around the shame that I hadn't yet managed to let go of?

In hindsight, I recognise this as impostor syndrome. I know that the way I was thinking of my asexuality – as if it was a kind of diagnosis I would have to live with and try to live my life *in spite of* – did not come from me but from what I had been told about what asexuality meant. This shame came from the way that everyone around me for most of my life spoke about sex, and sexual and romantic relationships: as a fundamental human need, something without which I could not be fully human.

As you can probably guess, I did end up signing the contract. Part of me must have known that not only did I want to write this book, I *needed* to write it, because I needed to unlearn all the things I had been told about myself that made me ashamed of who I was. I needed to write this book because I knew this project could benefit the community – *my* community – and I knew the community was "out there" somewhere, but I didn't really believe it. I knew other people "shared my experiences" and that those experiences were "valid", but again, I didn't really believe it. I was still feeling alone in my ace-ness.

What I hadn't yet realised, what I wouldn't fully understand until I'd actually started writing, was that many, *many* of us feel exactly as I did. In that sense, my insecurity itself made me a good fit to write it, because it united me with countless others who were like me and felt the same. It created a tension in me, a drive to try to use this book to help my community and myself, not from a place of peace and self-acceptance, but very much from a place of need.

Many people on the asexual spectrum spend much of their lives believing they are the only ones like this – the only person in the world who doesn't want a boyfriend, who isn't comfortable having sex with their partner even though they've been together for years, who can't understand how others recognise that ineffable spark, romantic love. I myself spent years waiting to feel *it* – even though no one ever really told me what *it* was – and believing there was something wrong with me when I didn't.

We come to think of ourselves as abnormal, sick, broken or missing something. We are told that there is no way to be as we are and still be happy, and therefore we need to be fixed. Lots of us don't get the chance I got and spend their whole lives thinking this. Thinking that in order to have a place in society, in order to be deserving of love, we have to change ourselves, sometimes painfully.

What's become clear to me while I've written this book, reading and listening to the experiences of people like me, is that none of this is our fault. There's nothing about being asexual, aromantic, demi or grey-a that is inherently bad, wrong, sick or broken. I want to take pains to tell anyone reading this who has felt broken, or ashamed, or alone, because of who they are: there is nothing wrong with you, and though you may feel alone, you are not.

We feel shame because we're living in a world that hasn't yet made room for us. We're erased and marginalised because asexuality, aromanticism, demi and grey-a identities challenge the status quo. Any refusal by any person to abide by the role society dictates for them puts – has always put – them at risk of being pathologised, dismissed, demonised or otherwise disempowered or rendered invisible. This is hard-won knowledge, and it's come at the end of more than two years of studying, listening and learning, of speaking to people who were like me, finding them among friends and people I admire, of reading words people like me had written. I hope that by sharing some of that knowledge in the form of this book, I'll make it a little easier for the next person to go through what I went through.

In her book *Ace*, journalist Angela Chen discusses[1] the way our sex drive and the impulse to form romantic partnerships, raise children and build families may have roots in evolution – they reflect our instinctual drive to reproduce and ensure the survival of our offspring. Sex, reproduction and coupledom are politically charged, too: throughout human history, who is allowed to have sex with whom, who is allowed to marry and have children and with whom are things that those in power, be it the State, church or king, have tried to control through laws and taboos.

In this light, it's possible to see how human sexuality and romantic love have come to be *seen* as organic, universal impulses that every human has. Under these conditions, asexuality and its spectrum are met with disbelief: "You mean you've never had sex *ever*?!", "But don't you want to find *the one*?" Our existence is erased: AK, an asexual aromantic woman I spoke to, told me that, "For a long time Polish Wikipedia showed that 'A' in LGBTQIA+ stands for 'ally'." There are social and legal repercussions, as well: aside from the fact that couples are more likely to be able to afford and be approved for mortgages, for example, sex is often codified into law. LL, who is ace, informed me:

> There are legal things to take into account when you are a-spec. For example, in France, a woman was considered at fault in her divorce because she didn't have sex with her husband. We should have a conversation about what legal texts (notably marriage laws) say about sex and how it impacts a-spec people. About rape between spouses, and "marriage duties", that sort of thing.

We are also living in a world, at least in the West, where human sexuality has been medicalised,[2] and where our identities have been defined by outsiders, not ourselves.

This is thanks in large part to the efforts of "sexologists" like William Masters and Virginia Johnson, who in the 1950s developed what they called the "human sexual response cycle". Through laboratory observations of anatomy and behaviour, they sought to map out the physiological stages of human sexual arousal and intercourse. The major upshot of their research was that they developed a clinical approach to treating what they decided were sexual dysfunctions; in other words, anyone whose sexual "response" didn't fit with the model they had derived from a small sample of mostly white, middle-class, heterosexual married couples. Thanks to the effort of the sexologists, asexuality was transformed into a formal diagnosis: "hypoactive sexual desire disorder"[3,4].

Today's medical institutions are structured in a way that disallows the possibility of asexuality – or any sexuality that doesn't fit the narrow, medicalised picture of sexual-romantic behaviour – existing in its own right. Asexuality is not allowed to exist as an identity, or as a natural, harmless human variation, but only as an illness to be fixed.

Like the Black and transgender[5] communities before them, the fraught history between biomedical science and the ace community has led to a deep sense of mistrust. Most of the ace spectrum people I spoke to while writing this book told me that they were not open about their identities with doctors or medical practitioners for fear that doctors would, as EF, who is asexual and aromantic, puts it, "react negatively and try to 'cure' me". But there are contexts when disclosure – of sexual activity, at least – becomes compulsory. A handful of my interviewees recalled times when, upon disclosure, health professionals in various disciplines had assumed they were mentally or physically ill or in distress simply by virtue of their asexuality. RK related the following incident:

> I was once offered therapy when I went to have the contraceptive implant replaced. The nurse seemed very concerned that I was a woman in my 30s who'd never had a cervical exam because I wasn't sexually active. She didn't seem to take my aceness as enough of an explanation. It didn't much matter in the end. (I have the implant to stop super-heavy periods.)

BH, when asked what medical professionals could do to support a-spec people, said:

> It's not an ace-spec-specific thing, but believing me when I assure them I'm not pregnant would be so nice. As a woman in my twenties, pregnancy is assumed to be a strong possibility and doctors do not believe me when I tell them I've never had penetrative sex (and I haven't had *any* sex in five years).

BH went on to add, "My therapist treated my lack of desire and interest in partnership as a symptom of depression, and although it wasn't a big focus, it still felt like my orientation needed to be cured."

Ace people are regularly offered drugs, therapy and hormone treatments,[6] all regardless of whether we are actually hurting or in distress[7] – in many cases these diagnoses are motivated by profit margins more than the wellbeing of the patient.[8] Never is it accepted that we might just *be* the way we are. This medicalisation bleeds over into real life as well: one 2012 study found that of all marginalised sexualities, asexual people were "evaluated more negatively, viewed as less human, and less valued as contact partners, relative to heterosexuals and other sexual minorities".[9]

Most asexual, aromantic, demi and grey-a people live in a world where not wanting sex or romance, or not wanting them enough or at the right time, is considered wrong and shameful. Even our ability to be seen as human is contingent on our willingness to conform to other people's sexual and romantic expectations of us.

But we're marginalised not because there's anything wrong with us – though many of us do have needs that differ from accepted norms – but because the very fact of our existence questions the legitimacy of established structures, from capitalism,[10] monogamy and the nuclear family[11] to white supremacy[12] and heteropatriarchy: happy aroace women with no interest in settling down and having children give the lie to the lesson young girls are taught, that they should seek fulfilment in aspirations of having a husband and family. Committed, loving relationships that don't involve reproductive, PiV sex – be they allo same-sex relationships or asexual relationships – threaten the myth that the nuclear family is the bedrock of society.

My own refusal to seek out conventional sexual-romantic relationships, my valuing of friendship over other kinds of love – and indeed my decision to change my appearance to better reflect my own understanding of my gender – is a kind of resistance to everything I had been told about myself since birth.

And just like with binary gender, it's also possible to see *past* politics and evolutionary coding, past the politically motivated myths we've been told about ourselves, and to understand asexuality, aromanticism and all the spectrum of identities for what they really are: nothing more than different ways to be human.

One of the most profound lessons I learned over the course of writing this book was that, while people who don't feel sexual attraction or who don't fall in romantic love are seen as fundamentally "other", inherently different from "normal" people, I don't think that's true. Our experiences are not so different from the "average" person's. After all, what is average? Who decides? Who gets to be counted?

It seems pretty clear that the traditional picture – media-driven and politically motivated – of love, sex, coupledom, of somehow finding your soulmate in a haystack of seven billion, with sexual, emotional and domestic compatibility paving the way towards a happily ever after, doesn't actually work for most people. After two years of listening to people talk about their experiences, that aspirational storyline – fed to us from the first moment we're old enough to watch Disney movies – seems almost laughable. How can we know what we want, when TV, advertising and medical science muddy the water so much it becomes opaque?

This is why I'm writing this book: because despite the fact that ace-spectrum people are increasingly telling our stories, and fighting for rights and visibility, there is still so much pressure for us to hide our identities. They are hidden even from ourselves. We're taught as young people to see ourselves as normatively sexual and desiring, and any step away from that norm requires disclosure. We internalise shame because no one tells us anything different is possible.

I'm writing this book because I want to join the conversation, helping to change the definitions we've been given that define us as lacking, refusing or missing out. And when you look at our actual experiences, the picture becomes more complicated. Indeed, many of the asexual people who shared their stories with me said they *do* have sex; many even enjoy it. Many of the aromantic people I spoke to still enjoyed the trappings of romance, even if they didn't feel romantically attracted to others. And in the end, sex and romance are not the only important things to fill a life with.

It seems to me that rather than missing out on anything, ace, aro, demi and grey-a people are finding *new* ways to love, new and alternative relationships that suit our needs, new ways to live our lives. Even the most common definition of asexuality, a simple lack of sexual attraction for others, is not how many of the people I spoke to define it for themselves.

I no longer want to start every discussion around our identities from a place of lack; I want to add my voice to the voices of the a-spec activists, writers, researchers and artists who are exploring positive, radically different ways of thinking about ourselves and our communities.

Over the course of this book, I'll be challenging some of the myths that a-spec people have been told about ourselves, and the myths that we have had to create in the name of visibility. I argue that asexuality and aromanticism are not really separate identities but are categories with porous, blurry boundaries, that overlap with allo experiences. I'll explore the positive, unique perspectives of asexual spectrum people, the ways we experience love and the relationships and spaces we are claiming for ourselves.

I'll discuss the language we've created to describe ourselves and our ways of being in the world, the history of our community and how it came to be the shape it is today, as well as the communities we've fought alongside in our efforts to achieve equality – and sometimes come into conflict with.

In my quest for a more positive portrayal of my community, I'll explore what our lived experiences look like today, the relationships that are most important to us, the different ways we relate to intimacy and sex, and the perspectives that are sometimes lost in mainstream discussions of asexuality, such as those at the intersection of a-spec identity and race, gender, neurodivergence and disability.

Finally, I'll talk about the most personal part of this book for me, which has been finding joy in being asexual and grey-aromantic. Writing this book proved to me that my asexuality is just another part of who I am, like my trans gender, like my neurodivergence, that being this way is something to celebrate, and that I'm not alone in it.

Perhaps ironically, realising I'm not alone has made me more comfortable with being on my own. Now that I know I can be ace and still have love, companionship, family and community, I also know I can stand on my own two feet. I don't need anyone else just because society tells me I do, and I'm more determined than ever to live life on my own terms.

I hope that by writing this book I can help take the perception of loneliness that clings to our community and replace it with a sense of celebration, togetherness, connection and family feeling. I want to bring together a volume, in every sense of the word, of a-spec voices, to challenge the idea that we are so few and far between as to be unworthy of notice. The chance that someone reading this book might encounter something that resonates with them, that offers them space and language for self-acceptance, is reason enough to write.

Since beginning this book I've begun, probably self-indulgently, to think of a-spec people like stars scattered across the night sky. Each of us is brilliant, interesting and unique, and though it may seem like any one of us is alone in the vacuum of space, the longer you look, the more of us you realise there are. And while we might be separated by physical distance, we're certainly not alone.

Visibility

The first time I saw an asexual, aromantic person portrayed positively in a piece of media, it was on the blogging site Tumblr, in a piece of *Les Misérables* fanfiction (yes, really). I read a lot of fanfiction in those days, but this one, a bare few thousand words, sticks in my memory because the character, whom the author had interpreted as asexual and aromantic, was not portrayed as sad, depressed, a loser or socially inept – in other words they weren't portrayed like every other ace character I'd encountered. Instead, they were the central figure in a group of friends, and what they seemed to lack in sexual or romantic feelings was replaced by other passions: this character's ideals were portrayed as the all-encompassing passion of their life, in the same way that so many characters have a single romantic love that defines them.

I was at university, in my late teens or maybe even my twenties, and I was Very Online in the way that so many babyqueers are before they find their communities in real life. If I hadn't been, I'd never have stumbled across this fanfiction. It might have been years before the idea that being aroace was anything but a sad, depressing, doomed existence was made real to me.

Part of the reason I spent so much time on the internet back then was because I took it for granted that meeting an out, a-spec person in real life was not a possibility. I spent a good few hours a day online, talking to friends, reading blogs or consuming pop culture – an amount of time that today feels totally unthinkable. Tumblr was a strange, stressful, often unpleasant place in many ways, which is why I eventually stopped using it, but it was also one of the few places where I didn't have to explain myself or justify my existence.

It's been proven that visibility matters: seeing yourself reflected in a piece of even fictional media allows you to envision new possibilities for yourself. So why did it take wading into the depths of the internet before I could see someone like me portrayed positively?

At the time of writing, I've only come across a few pieces of positive a-spec representation, and I've had to work hard to scrape together even the paltry list I include at the end of this book. Representation in nonfictional media, too, is still nascent. Most of the writing about our experiences, save a few notable exceptions, is still in the form academic books and articles.

It took years for me to see anyone who was openly *like me* living their life proudly and happily, or accomplishing anything of note. I had always figured that if I could have a career, be successful, fulfilled and happy, it would be *in spite* of my being a-spec. This feeling persisted until I started encountering the work of out a-spec writers, researchers and activists such as Yasmin Benoit, Angela Chen, David Jay and Alice Oseman – to whom I will always be indebted.

We've come a long way from the sensationalised, daytime talk-show interviews of the early 2000s, where asexuality was displayed as a scandalous oddity to entertain an allosexual audience. This is thanks in large part to the efforts of those in our community who have not been able to see themselves reflected in existing portrayals – especially people of colour and those from outside the Anglophone West. But there is still work to do. For a community whose existence is still regularly denied, for people who may spend years thinking there's no one else out there like them, visibility is all the more important.

There is strength in numbers. There's also healing, joy, companionship and connection in numbers. For many of us, that moment of realisation – of finally understanding that there are other people out there who have gone through what we're going through, in numbers never imagined – is life-changing.

As it turns out, aromantic, asexual, demi and grey-a people are everywhere.

While I'm writing this book, the 2020 Ace Census survey data has just been released, with over 15,000 people taking part. AVEN – the Asexual Visibility and Education Network, founded by David Jay in 2001 – has over 135,000 members.[1] New books are coming out every month about a-spec experiences and with a-spec characters. Yasmin Benoit, a Black aroace model and activist, has done shoots for *Vogue*, *Cosmopolitan*, *Teen Vogue* and *Glamour*.

When I first started writing this book, people reached out to me from the UK, the USA, Ireland, Canada and Australia, but also Spain, Malaysia, France, Germany, Pakistan, Belgium, Japan, Denmark, The Netherlands, Norway, Poland, Italy, Argentina, Finland, Switzerland, Russia, Hong Kong, Brazil and Lithuania – and these were just those who were able to contact me over the internet, in English, and who used these English-language terms to describe themselves.

This realisation – that we are everywhere, that I've always been surrounded by a-spec people, even among my close friends, though I didn't realise it – was deeply profound and healing.

Over and over, when asked, "How did it make you feel, finding out that there were other people like you out there?", the a-spec people I spoke to expressed relief, reassurance and belonging, and a lifting of the burdens of shame and impending, permanent solitude.

> I always assumed that if there were people like me out there, they had some kind of physical or mental illness or some past trauma keeping them from being "normal". It's such a relief to have words for what I am other than "something is wrong with me". BH

> Amazing. I hadn't entirely believed I was different before then, I'd just thought no one really got attracted, but the feeling that maybe I was the one who was different had slowly been creeping up on me for the previous year. It was so good to hear that yes, I was different, but that difference was perfectly okay, and I wasn't alone in it. LM

Interviewee LH describes a sense of "soul-shaking relief. I was not broken, I was not weird, I was just not in the majority. It lifted so much of the pressure and shame I'd been putting on myself." EP, who is bisexual and demi- or aromantic, says she felt "like a weight had been lifted. Relieved. I could stop stressing about how defective I was. Because I had felt defective." JTS describes his greysexuality as a missing piece in the puzzle of his identity:

> I think it was gradual, but I knew since I was a child. The easiest thing was to find out I was not straight. The second easiest was knowing that I liked men. Finally, when I found out about the [ace] spectrum, I knew I found the missing piece of that puzzle that my sexual orientation seemed to be. It was so relieving as I could now describe and refer to that part of my identity with

> exact words. I was about 18 or 19 years old… I think it was one of the best feelings I've ever had. I finally could be honest with myself and live as what I've always been and didn't dare to show.

For JTS, and many others, the moment when it finally "clicks", when you stop feeling defective and start feeling like part of a big family, isn't just the end of self-doubt or shame but also a necessary piece of self-knowledge. Discovering the a-spec community, and fully coming to understand that there's nothing wrong with being a-spec, means fully allowing yourself to exist.

So why does it take so many of us years, even decades, to come to this understanding? The answer to that question is tied fundamentally to visibility. As I've said before, if you can't see something and name it, it can't exist for you. Without seeing that there are other asexual and aromantic people out there – *whole* people who look like us, not caricatures or stereotypes – there's no way to see ourselves as anything other than broken.

I asked my interviewees about the barriers they encountered that prevented them from discovering their a-spec identities. One of the most common answers was a lack of inclusive sex education. Sex ed in schools, even when it allows for the existence of LGBT+ people, tends to have as a basic assumption that students, especially teenagers, *will* want to couple up and have sex, and the main concern is that they should do it safely.

Many recounted attending religious schools that taught abstinence-only programmes. And even these programmes tend to be based on an assumption that human beings are sexual by nature, with the caveat that these basic, universal sexual urges must be curtailed until the socially sanctioned coupledom of marriage – in fact, abstinence-only programmes exist entirely *because* of this assumption.

Whatever the ideological foundation of a given programme,

in many ways sex ed creates an *expectation* that young people will pair up and explore sex – in more or less healthy, more or less clandestine ways. This expectation can quickly slide into obligation, which creates problems for students who *don't* feel sexual attraction or who have no desire for a romantic partner.

Paired with the closed and often privacy-less environment of a high or secondary school, social expectations or peer pressure can push young a-specs into unsafe or unwanted situations. AB, who knew she was aroace but didn't realise it was a real or acceptable thing to be until she was 20 years old, is keenly aware of how expectations around sex and relationships can put young people in danger. She describes her first relationship as a teenager (the emphasis is AB's):

> We became close friends at that time and started dating which I *agreed to because I thought that was the normal way of doing things (you know the typical "becoming good friends with someone of a different gender means you will date them eventually" bullshit).* At that time, I didn't realise that I wasn't interested in dating. I knew right away that I wasn't "in love" with him but I thought these feelings would come along eventually (I, again, thought "forcing" myself into the relationship long enough would make it work). I started becoming extremely uncomfortable in the relationship, even though he was super nice and caring towards me. I knew that I wouldn't be happy in the relationship, so we broke up.
>
> I still – to this day – appreciate his behavior because I know how damaging it could have become for both of us: for me if he had forced me (or if I had forced myself more) into the relationship and certain actions that he assumed I would be okay with; and for him if the relationship had turned toxic due to miscommunication (since I didn't know I was aroace yet so

he couldn't have known either). I'm glad we actually broke up on good terms and no one got hurt.

AB explicitly links her experiences as a teen to the social norms around relationships that are beginning to be learned at that age: the expectation that a boy and a girl who are friends will date eventually, the idea that love grows with familiarity and that forcing oneself to continue in an unwanted relationship will make those feelings magically appear.

If AB had had access to the knowledge that asexuality and aromanticism exist when she was a teenager, if she'd learned about them in sex ed or in the media or from her parents, she might have felt more comfortable asserting herself, staying friends instead of allowing the relationship to morph into a romantic one, and saving them both heartache and potential trauma.

Of course, it's not always as simple as just learning the word "asexual" or "aromantic" and everything instantly clicking into place. Even in cases where nascent a-specs do learn words like demisexual or aromantic, there's still a considerable leap from there to self-acceptance, or even just having the confidence to claim the label for themselves. Yasmin Benoit, in an interview for *AZ Magazine*[2] mentions a lag between learning the word asexual – a basic description of her experiences, a word some strangers on the internet labelled themselves with – and realising that it *meant something*. She says, "I was like, okay, I have a word. But then I was also like, no one else knows or cares about this? So, it really wasn't actually that helpful." It wasn't until Yasmin met other aroace people, especially other Black aroace people, in real life that she fully believed there were others out there like her, with full lives, who were part of a *community*, a movement, something to be proud of. This is part of why she created the hashtag and movement #thisiswhatasexuallookslike:

> Because that was one of the things that I noticed, when I would be on social media trying to find out what is this community, you can find a lot of blocks of text, but you can't see many faces. And I think that it's quite a unique experience for the asexual community, where you could literally go through life and not meet another openly asexual person... I thought that it would be helpful for people to just be able to actually see faces.

Again, visibility is the key here: because Yasmin didn't have any positive asexual representation or role models to look up to – only strangers on the internet, if not totally faceless then almost always white – it took that much longer for her to be able to claim "aroace" for herself in a positive way.

A number of people I've spoken to have also mentioned that same lag, between learning the words and claiming them for themselves, or even between learning the words and realising they were relevant to their own experience. An ace person who'd been in a sexual relationship in the past might have a harder time accepting their own asexuality if all they'd ever seen were so-called "gold star" aces: otherwise-normative, asexual people who had never had sex. Another aspect of this "gold star" narrative, that claims ace people "can love like anyone else" – a necessary talking point to push back against the idea that ace people are soulless robots – has still ended up narrowing the visible picture of the community and alienating people who don't feel normative romantic love.

In this way, a lot of early ace activism, which ironically focused so much on visibility, has inadvertently contributed to the erasure of some parts of the community. Aromantic allosexual people, like the anonymous aro whose feedback I'll talk about in the next chapter, as well as asexuals who are ill or disabled, or who just don't look like the aces on TV, may find it that much harder to see themselves in the community and make their voices heard.

There are external barriers to visibility as well, which mean that certain a-spec people are not able to make their voices heard in the same way as the aces doing TV interviews and writing articles and books.

In a 2021 AceCon panel of North American Indigenous aces,[3] Johnnie Jae, an Otoe-Missouria and Choctaw journalist and advocate, made the point that not everyone has *access* to the visible a-spec community, which is so online and urban focused. Many Native American communities lack reliable access to the internet and rely on alternative forms of communication, such as radio, printed newspapers or running.[4] People living in rural areas, or on reservations as many Indigenous North Americans do, may not have the same connectivity as the average urban dweller – but internet access is often taken as a given when discussing the circumstances of younger a-spec people.

This lack of access may create a self-fulfilling prophecy, a kind of invisibility feedback loop: unable to access the specialised a-spec language used on forums and blogging sites, and unable to see a full picture of the community's diversity, Indigenous a-spec people may find it hard to see each other and to make themselves visible – especially since the Indigenous community is already so overwhelmingly invisible[5] within American society. Sitting at this intersection adds a layer of complexity onto an already complex identity. The overwhelming perception of whiteness and Westernness – and online-ness – of popular images of asexuality means that Indigenous aces may struggle to, as Johnnie Jae puts it, be "seen and understood".

So the more visibly diverse the a-spec community is, the more likely it is that an a-spec person who is not yet out will see something that resonates with them. Because of course, it's not enough to just see someone describe a similar experience of romance or sexuality. If that person looks nothing like you, it's easy enough to just think, "Well, that's alright for *them*, but it's not for me." But if you see an a-spec person from the same cultural background as you, with the same disability as you or from the same country or community as you, it's much easier for you to picture yourself in their shoes.

This is why events like the Indigenous Aces panel and articles by a-specs from marginalised backgrounds are so important within the larger conversation around a-spec issues. Those of us already here must make sure that our community, which so prides itself on inclusivity and collaboration, is welcoming to everyone.

Most asexual visibility activism so far has been about convincing outsiders that we exist. But our fight for liberation should not be about assimilation to an allo norm, or convincing the majority that "we're just like you". Instead we should be celebrating the fact that we *are* different: showing the wide breadth of experiences encompassed by the word "a-spec" and asserting that no matter who you are or where you come from, you have a place in the community if you want it. This is why movements like #thisiswhatasexuallookslike are so groundbreaking: not because they prove to allosexuals that we exist, but because they prove it to *ourselves*.

Discussion questions

1. Thinking about the a-spec (or asexual) community, what was your "mental picture" of it before starting this book? Did it look a certain way? Did it consist of certain types of people?
2. Are there parts of your identity – cultural, sexual, gender, national and so on – that are more or less apparent to outsiders? Are there parts that are invisible? Why?
3. What are the places and contexts in which you feel most seen? Are these different for different facets of your identity?

Who Are We?

I love words. I love language. I've always been fascinated by the many weird and wonderful ways humans have found to express themselves. At university, I spent five years studying language, especially the ways languages change, adapting and evolving to fit new circumstances and concepts. But it wasn't until I wrote this chapter that it occurred to me I might be interested in language change because I have a personal stake in it, as well.

Language changes because society changes. And it's only because of social change in the last ten or twenty years that I can put into words the way that I experience sexuality and gender. When I found the terms "asexual", "grey-aromantic" and "transgender", it was like a door opened: I suddenly had the words to talk about how I was feeling – words other people could understand. I was able to be visible, not only to others but to myself, in a way I never could before. And even if it took some time for me to embrace these words and claim them in coming out, I could never have done so at all without first having the language.

I've tried out various terms over the years: nonbinary, demiromantic, agender, genderqueer. I don't always keep them – queer vocabulary is always being updated, and my feelings change too. But with each new word I find, explore, keep or discard, I understand myself a little better.

In order to talk about something, in order to explore it and celebrate it, you first need to name it. As a nonbinary, neurodivergent, grey-aroace person, I rely on words like these to help me understand myself and articulate how I exist in the world.

Many of the terms used by the asexual-spectrum community to describe ourselves are relatively new, having been collaboratively developed over the last few decades by members of the community themselves, mostly on forums – especially AVEN – and social media and blogging platforms like Tumblr.

But the language of our community isn't completely new: asexuality, as a word or concept, is by no means a modern invention. Asexual people have actually been identifying as such for as long as we have been categorising people based on "sexual orientation",[1] and asexuality has at various times, especially in the context of the gay rights movement, been considered in its own right alongside L, G, B and T.[2,3] There are archive photos from the 1970s of young feminists standing in front of a sign inviting the viewer to "choose your own label", with "asexual" written clearly alongside "bi" and "lesbian". In 1981, an ace woman wrote to feminist magazine *Heresies*[4] expressing concern that asexuals were not being represented in the LGBT movement, and that asexuality, "is seen as a negativity, a lack, an expression of the incompleteness of a human being".

But even if all of our words were invented last week, why does it matter? It's natural for language to change and evolve over time, and as society's understanding of sexuality, gender, desire and attraction have changed, so have the words used by the a-spec community to describe feelings that have always existed.

Old terms fall out of favour and others are coined or cobbled together, and in the internet age this can happen at lightning speed. A single person with a blog might create a new word that quickly proliferates throughout the community – the now hugely popular word "demisexual" was coined in 2006 by AVEN user sonofzeal.[5] New words spark into existence and float through the air: sometimes they catch alight and sometimes they extinguish.

The way our vocabulary has been built over time through collaboration speaks volumes about us as a community. In their essay "Radical Identity Politics",[6] gender and race scholar Erica Chu discusses the highly precise and inclusive vocabulary that has crystallised around the ace-spectrum community. Communities and spaces like AVEN, Tumblr and Reddit are conducive to non-hierarchical uses of language. Chu says:

> AVEN has succeeded in creating an environment of transparency and plurality that the dominant institutions involved in the theoretical development of other identity groups were not able to replicate.

In other words, the very fact that our community has mainly been built in online forums, where anyone present is able to contribute their ideas, means that the vocabulary and concepts we use are truly reflective – though of course with the caveat that not everyone has access to that space – of who we are and what we want.

As a rule, on these platforms no single person present has a say over what means what – even words' creators can see their creations go in unexpected directions. There are no hard-and-fast definitions: even for the "big" words like asexual and aromantic, each one is *explicitly* acknowledged to mean different things to different people.

This flexibility is a strength. In many ways the "microlabels" I'll be exploring in the next chapter, often derided by people outside our community for being "made up", are radical acts of defiance. For a group of people constantly accused of being "special snowflakes", and constantly having their experiences of marginalisation diminished as "internet identities",[7] creating a secret language – coining neologisms to use amongst ourselves, to get at specific and difficult-to-articulate shades of experience not admitted by mainstream understandings of sexuality and attraction – can be empowering. In creating new words, proliferating them and stubbornly using them even in the face of ridicule when their uniqueness and obscurity is used against us, we're exercising what Chu calls "individual agency in negotiating one's relationship to oneself and others"[8]: we're taking back some of the power denied to us. By making our language as inclusive as possible, we make space for those who have been refused the power to name themselves.

But as a marginalised community gains visibility and begins to fight more openly for social and legal recognition, there is also mounting pressure to be able to explain ourselves clearly and consistently – to present a unified front – to outsiders. Under these conditions, standardised vocabulary emerges whether anyone intends it to or not. Definitions are agreed upon, and the difference between words as pure descriptors of lived experience and words as political tools becomes clear.

What follows are the most common terms that the people I spoke to used to describe themselves, and their most common definitions. But keep in mind that a definition I give here won't necessarily work for everyone who uses that word. I've tried to rely as much as possible on the words that the people I spoke to used to talk about themselves, but I'm not trying to dictate how anyone names or describes their experience.

Asexual

This is by far the most common term used in the community. Of the 39 people I spoke to in depth, 26 described themselves as asexual, be that alongside another identity like a-, demi- or panromantic, or just "asexual" on its own. In the basic demographic information provided by the 160 people who reached out to me to register their interest in the project, the word "asexual" appears 120 times. In the 2020 Ace Census, 65 per cent of the 15,131 respondents answered "asexual" to the question "Which of the following sexual orientation labels do you most closely identify with?", with other answers including "questioning", aromantic and demisexual, "microlabels" like aegosexual, or leaving the question blank, and other questions asking about "secondary" identities and identity history.

Asexuality is usually defined as a lack of sexual attraction towards, or a lack of desire for sexual intercourse with, another person. As KL, one of the people I spoke to in more depth, says, "You know that thing where you look at someone and go, that person is hot? Yeah, that just doesn't happen with me." DC echoes them, rather facetiously: "You know how sometimes you're walking down the street and you see someone walking towards you and you *don't* want to have sex with them? It's like that but all the time." CF, who is asexual and on the aromantic spectrum, uses a food metaphor:

> Sexual attraction is like wanting pizza, and in a world where almost everybody wants pizza (each one a different kind of pizza, but still pizza). I do not have any desire to eat pizza. This doesn't mean I cannot eat pizza, or that if I try it I wouldn't like it, but still I never experience the desire to eat pizza.

Not everyone I spoke to defined their asexuality in terms of sexual *attraction*, but everyone who called themself "ace" or "asexual" included something about not wanting or feeling the need for sex with another person. NT said, "I can recognise others as both sexually and romantically attractive, but have no desire to have a sexual relationship."

This doesn't necessarily mean not wanting relationships at all, though. As BH says, "Many asexuals, myself included, want to date and get married and have sex although the sex is a much less important part of the equation for many of us, myself included." Indeed, a good number of the asexuals I spoke to said they were married or in romantic or queerplatonic (see the "microlabels" section for a definition) relationships of some kind. And even those who said they didn't want "relationships" still tended to deeply value friendships and family bonds; none of us are what you might call islands.

Asexual people can be sex repulsed or sex ambivalent, but we can also enjoy sex and be happy to have sex with a trusted partner. As LL says, "I have libido and enjoy sexual activities, but I never feel sexually attracted to anyone, in any circumstances." And pretty much all of us, even the most personally sex repulsed, are at the very least *politically* sex positive. I'll go into more detail about our experiences with and attitudes toward sex towards the end of the book.

Ace

Because of its origins within scientific and biomedical contexts, the word "asexual" still carries some clinical flavour. It's still often associated with non- (or sub-) human organisms. As a teenager, still very much self-conscious about my emergent (a)sexuality, I endured jokes, even by my friends, about how I would reproduce by budding.

Because of these associations (and for convenience and the potential for wordplay), "asexual" is often shortened to "ace". For many people, "ace" means the same as the lack of sexual attraction described above, but ace (and "asexual", for that matter!) is also often used as an umbrella term – in the same way I use "a-spec" – to describe a whole constellation of related, overlapping and adjacent identities.

Because the terminology is always changing and adapting, and some parts of the community may use the language differently than others, the use of "ace" and "asexual" as umbrella terms can be a source of tension within the community. Our collectivist and self-determined usage of terms can both empower us and create conflict between us.

Many people I spoke to also used ace or asexual not necessarily as an umbrella for the community as a whole, but to describe a personal experience of sexuality that was nebulous or in flux, or that a person wasn't ready to explore too deeply at that moment. Many people don't feel the need to share – or even discover – the *precise* nature of their sexuality or way of experiencing attraction, and many of these people use "ace" as a convenient way to align themselves with the community while not digging too deep. HBJ, in describing how she arrived at the words she uses, said:

> I usually just say I'm on the ace spectrum. Whether I'm completely asexual, grey, demi or what, I haven't completely determined even after a couple decades knowing I'm in there somewhere, but I also don't care too much to pin it down. Being "ace" is enough... I decided not to dig too deep into trying to pin down a specific term.

Some people may describe themselves one way with a-spec friends, one way with strangers and one way in institutional settings: context determines what we are comfortable sharing and how much we feel the need to explain.

Words like asexual might only be useful when a boundary is crossed or community building is necessary: KL, for example, usually only uses the word "ace" or "asexual" "if someone tries to make a sexual joke about me, or if I'm disclosing to help another ace person understand their identity". For some people, such as IJ, the word asexual means "not being attracted to anyone", but "in a more explanatory way than an identity way". Not everyone I spoke to – in fact hardly anyone – had only one word to describe, or even give a static idea of, their identity: JK says, "I use grey-aromantic asexual. Or bi-oriented aroace. It depends on what feels better for me to say at the given time."

The more people I spoke to, the more I realised that the set definitions, and the boundaries we might draw between and around each of our words, were more a convenient shorthand than reality. Identity and desire are not static. Our feelings and understandings of ourselves change over time, and acknowledging this is one of the ways in which the a-spec community is at the forefront of thought around sexuality and attraction. There are as many ways to describe and define asexuality as there are asexual people, and yet each of these experiences is, by definition, still an asexual one.

Aro(mantic)

This was the second most commonly encountered word while I was writing this book – 51 of 160 people described themselves this way in my initial contact form. Compared to asexual, the exact meaning of aromantic, and where it interlocks with other a-spec orientations, is a little harder to pin down – or rather, it is difficult to pin down for different reasons.

Many people described aromanticism, similarly to asexuality, in terms of a lack of romantic attraction, but just as often it was described as not feeling the need to form romantic attachments. EP, who is bisexual and demi- or aromantic, says: "I've always been sexually attracted to all genders. But I don't get interested in people. Or if I do, it's this once-in-a-decade feeling." AK, aroace, says: "I have no desire to form a romantic relationship." DE, also aroace, said that when people ask her to explain her identity, "I'll just say that I'm really happy being single and I'm not interested in dating." EF on the other hand described being aroace, realising the aromantic aspect of their identity, in terms of the way being in a romantic relationship would make them feel:

> I would consistently feel uncomfortable with the way I felt that I had to behave when in a relationship (touching, PDA, prioritising your romantic partner, the general feeling of being stuck or trapped honestly).

I want to reiterate that the aromantic people I spoke to, even the aroace people, weren't necessarily uninterested in intimate attachments or connections of any kind. Many aromantic people described their ideal relationship as something intimate and caring but not romantic in the conventional sense. (In the chapters "What Is Love?" and "The Future of Relationships", I'll go into more detail about what these connections might look like.) And just like asexuality, context and personal history play a part as well: a relationship that an aromantic person describes as their ideal might still be perceived as romantic by someone else – as ever, our language is always ultimately self-applied.

At the same time, it's important to remember that intimate attachments need not be the be-all and end-all of humanity. A person's life still has value if they don't want these things or are more comfortable on their own. None of us are islands, but there is also no single bond or relationship that we must be in or seek out to qualify as human.

As I mentioned in the last chapter, some of the visibility activism around our community, especially early on, has necessitated simplification in order to get the message across. In a similar way to how early gay and lesbian activism focused on gay marriage rather than radical system change, we as a community have been obliged to repackage our experiences to make them intelligible to journalists and daytime TV talk-show hosts.

In order to be taken seriously on allo platforms, ace activists have had to challenge the notion that sex and sexual attraction specifically are universally healthy and natural. Part of this strategy has been the rhetoric of "we fall in love just like anyone else".[9] And just as in the LGBT community,[10] this pressure to assimilate, to prove that we are "otherwise normal" *despite* being asexual, leaves some members of our community behind.

So-called "gold star aces",[11] asexual but also usually white, cisgender and in a loving, committed heteroromantic relationship, are offered up as a counter to myths around asexuality: we can love, we're still human, we're not robots.

But where does this leave people who *don't* form romantic connections? Making the ability or desire to enter romantic relationships into an implicit entry requirement into the ranks of "functional" or "good" a-specs excludes a huge portion of our community. This may account for the fact that aroace people – who are both aromantic and asexual – made up 9 of the 40 people I spoke to in depth, compared to only one or two who were aromantic but *allosexual*, and out of the 51 aromantic people mentioned above, only 8 said they were aromantic *without also being asexual* (for example aro and bisexual like EP, or aromantic and demisexual).

I believe this apparent imbalance has to do with our community's political strategy of visibility activism, but also with the difficulty of disentangling sexual from romantic attraction, and romantic from other forms of attraction.

As I'll explore in the chapter titled "What Is Love?", a huge number of the people I spoke to mentioned not actually knowing what romantic attraction felt like, or not even being able to figure out what romance *is*. Lots of the aromantic people I spoke to said that they "enjoyed" romance, while not necessarily wanting it for themselves, at least not in that moment: LM, who is aroace, says, "Unlike sex, I actually want romance. I like reading a good romance novel, and I like listening to classic romantic songs."

Many aroace people I spoke to also mentioned a time lag between figuring out they were ace and figuring out they were aro because a lack of romantic feelings is a lot harder to identify than a lack of sexual attraction. AK, who is aroace, says that while figuring out she was asexual was fairly simple, "the 'aro' part was a little bit trickier. I was confused for quite a long time if this was what I felt."

The fact that romance is both ubiquitous and badly defined, making aromanticism a little harder to identify, may account for the fact that within the community people like EP, who are aromantic but *not* asexual, are often forgotten about or rendered invisible.

Very early in the process of writing this book, I received an anonymous response to my Google contact form from an aromantic person. They said that the early version of my "pitch" describing the scope and purpose of this book (which I billed as about "the experiences of asexual people"), made them uncomfortable, because I was (to quote them) "referring to this as a book about asexuality and then including aromanticism as if it's under the umbrella term of asexual". They went on to say:

> Aromanticism is so pushed aside and forgotten about already, even more so than asexuality is, and I feel like constantly as someone who's aro and ace spec, people are just like ah an ace.

I was shocked, not at the idea that someone would tell me off (I've been on the internet long enough not to be surprised), but that my usage of the word "asexual" as an umbrella term – a usage that I had encountered in both scholarship on and writing from within the a-spec community – could spark such a visceral reaction in someone. It had not been my intention to exclude or diminish any part of my community, so receiving this response felt as if the rug had been pulled out from under me.

This interaction was a reminder that, regardless of good intentions, when you're creating work using real people's experiences, those people's feelings are important. I realised I needed to step back and take a look at my own preconceptions before I could proceed.

For the reasons stated above, and because the word itself is slightly newer and less well established than asexuality, aromanticism was also less familiar to me as a concept, despite the fact that I myself am very much on the aromantic spectrum. The boundaries around the category of "aromantic" didn't seem as clear, and (at the time) I didn't think I had any personal experience with it. I knew I would need to tread carefully.

The first thing I did was to think hard about my own use of language: ace and even asexual *were* used as umbrella terms, but I had to admit that this did still end up centring asexuality – the sexual component of the experience – and made it much more difficult to talk about the *romantic* component, to be clear when I was discussing aromantic-but-not-necessarily-asexual experiences. This is surely a result of the way that society's understanding of romance as something that can exist apart from sexuality is still relatively new. This was a problem I'd had when reading a number of academic articles on the community: these authors tended to use only the word "asexual" to refer to a whole constellation of identities that may or may not be strictly *non-sexual*. They never seemed to articulate clearly *what* parts of the community they were talking about – or perhaps they weren't even aware that aro-allo people existed.

I had decided early on that this book would be useless if it wasn't as inclusive as possible, so I settled on "a-spec" – the word I use to refer to my community as a whole – throughout the book. It's technically short for "ace-" or "asexual-spectrum", but I like it because it highlights the "a-", the commonality between these sets of experiences, while allowing either one to occupy the foreground.

The next thing I wanted to do was to look, as far as I could, at aromantic experiences as *separate* from asexual ones. I wanted to look not only at the unique perspective of aromanticism and what it might teach us about desire and love but also at the unique challenges faced by aromantic people that alloromantic aces might not face.

One theme that emerged strongly from my reading about and interacting with aro people is that romantic love carries as much preconception and social baggage around it as sex does – though not necessarily of the same kind or in the same contexts. If sex is considered by mainstream society to be a normal and universal function of a healthy body or mind, then romance and romantic coupling – its sexual nature often left unsaid but still implied – is framed as a natural function of a healthy *personality*.

From the age we are old enough to read sanitised picture-book versions of fairy tales, we – especially those of us in the West, and especially those socialised as female – are introduced to the concept of romantic (hetero-, monogamous, reciprocal, committed) love as the pinnacle of human experience, the most wholesome and pure thing a person can feel: "They both lived happily ever after."

And while depictions of dysfunctional, abusive or unequal relationships do complexify this picture, the idea that romantic coupling is something to strive for, something to build your entire life around to the expense of everything else, persists. We are told constantly that we should try to find the perfect partner, we should try to stay with them faithfully for as long as we can, and any rocky patches or eventual breakups take on the whiff of moral failure.

So again, where does this leave people who don't "fall in love" in the way we expect them to? If forming idealised romantic attachments is the pinnacle of human achievement, what is there for people who don't form those attachments, who don't feel those feelings, but who are nonetheless undeniably human?

Over and over the people I spoke to mentioned pressure from family and friends, not necessarily to have sex, but to couple up, to "find the right person", to "settle down". When asked how she describes her aroace identity to someone who doesn't share it, AB says:

> I rarely say "I'm aromantic", not because it's any less important than my asexuality (in fact I feel like my aromanticism impacts my daily life more...), but rather because it involves more explaining and often more "having to justify myself to others".

Lots of the work done by asexual writers and activists has been around fighting back against the sexual "maturity narrative" that dictates that you "become an adult" when you have sex, that any intimate relationship must "progress" towards sexuality, and that a person who hasn't had sex "yet" is somehow naive, immature or innocent. This maturity narrative is often used against asexual people to frame us as naive, childlike or ignorant, to perpetuate the idea that we don't know our own minds and bodies, and, ultimately, to bar us from fully participating in our own political and social liberation.

But as I've spoken to more aromantic people, I've begun to see hints of another, parallel maturity narrative running alongside this one: the idea that "sex without love" isn't something that healthy, stable, fully grown people do. One-night stands are fine for your twenties or the odd midlife crisis, this narrative says, but you won't *really* be happy unless you ultimately end up in a committed romantic partnership. To do anything but spend your later decades sleeping every night beside the same person is treated, at least by mainstream media, as unbearably sad.

And while "romantic" immaturity can't as easily be used to take away our bodily agency, it still contributes to an atmosphere of shame and stigma for aromantic people – that feeling of brokenness and failure to live up to expectations around what it means to be a mature, fulfilled human being.

Of course, context is important, and romance and romantic bonds sit at an intersection of cultural, gendered and even economic norms and expectations. In communities where sex positivity is the norm and casual sex is a topic of conversation *de rigeur* – for example, in certain parts of the LGBTQ+ community – an asexual person might stick out like a sore thumb, attracting invasive questions or ridicule, while an aromantic person may be able to "pass" for allo. But in an environment where it's expected that a person of a certain age should be settling down and starting a family – like many religious communities or cultures where familial bonds come before all others – a person who has no desire to partner up may find it very hard to justify their existence.

I've found again and again while writing that different words take on different meanings in different contexts; there is no clear-cut way to describe who is marginalised and how, or who suffers and why. This is why arguments over whether a-spec people are "oppressed" enough to count as LGBT+ are utterly futile. This is also why I want to be as inclusive as I can in my word choice. In the end, it's *not* always about sex, and one of my goals for this book has actually been to de-centre sex, knocking it off its pedestal at the centre of our narratives. At the very least, using "a-spec", and being explicit when I'm talking about romantic experiences, is another way of doing so. Aromantic people *are* part of this community. And like so many others whose experiences have been marginalised within the community, it's important that their voices are heard.

Demi(sexual/romantic)

A few months ago, a group of friends and I went out for a drink after work. We were sitting around the table, tentatively enjoying our first beer out together since the pandemic began, and the conversation came around to the subject of dating. Friend A, a heterosexual woman, was expressing her frustration with the dating scene, discomfort with the fact that all the men she seemed to be matching with on the apps were only interested in sex; she couldn't imagine wanting to have sex with someone without knowing them really, really well – let alone on a first date. Dating was nearly impossible for her when what she wanted seemed so far removed from what her potential partners wanted: "I'm too picky!"

Friends B and C and I – a motley collection of queers – exchanged surreptitious glances. I spoke up, tentatively, suddenly afraid of being too aggressive with my suggestion.

"It kind of sounds like you're demisexual?"

"Oh."

My friend got quiet, and a thoughtful look came over her. Friend B – also demi – piped up in agreement, and we hastened to reassure friend A that, no pressure, but it might be worth looking into demisexuality. We steered the conversation elsewhere, not wanting to put Friend A on the spot.

Fast forward to a few weeks later, Friend A and I were eating lunch together, lying on a little slice of public grass that caught the sun – we were in the middle of a heatwave, which, watching the rain fall from the window over my desk, feels impossibly long ago. My friend said, "So I've been looking into demisexuality, and I think it fits." It was good, reassuring, my friend said, to know there was a name for how she felt, that there wasn't anything wrong with her, and – most importantly – that other people felt the same.

I rolled over to face her, trying to keep the grin off my face, trying to stop myself from shouting "WELCOME!" at her.

I mentioned that I'd been trying out OKCupid, which allowed you to select demi as your sexuality, and filter your potential matches to include ace-spectrum people only. We chatted a little bit more about it before the conversation moved on, but what I remember most strongly about that lunch hour is the warm glow of connection I felt, being able to bond with my friend over our shared experiences. I was pleased for her, because I knew how profound it had been for me, realising I wasn't alone in my asexuality. I felt deeply gratified to know it had been my suggestion that had led her to the same moment of enlightenment.

I've come to realise that people coming out to me is one of my favourite things. Not because I've gained some secret knowledge of them, but because of the idea that something I've said or written has helped them to discover a part of themselves. It's one of the most rewarding parts of being a writer, and of being a friend.

This sort of thing has happened several times – after sharing some materials for Asexual Awareness Week, another friend got in touch to say she'd been thinking she might be somewhere on the aromantic spectrum. This was someone I'd gotten "that vibe" from for a while but, again, I was wary of putting a label on her without her consent. Instead, I'd been talking about working on this book, and generally being open about my own experiences, when it came up in conversation. I trusted that, if the language and community were useful to my friend, she would come to them herself.

You can't force people to identify a certain way. That's one of the most frustrating things I see in aphobic rhetoric these days: the idea that we're, for example, "forcing" people to label themselves demisexual when in fact that's just "normal" sexuality, or that demisexual is just a "snowflake"[12] label for a common feeling.

Claims like this miss the point utterly. Our community, our language, were created entirely by and for the people for whom they are useful. We offer up these words, tentatively, on the chance that they will resonate, that whoever hears them will find something they need.

Personal history and life context will determine whether being demi is a point of pain for someone, and marginalisation may be the push that causes someone to seek out language to describe their experience and community to shelter in. A-spec community and language have always been – and I suspect always will be – self-determining and self-applied.

That's why visibility is so important. The proof is in the pudding: just look at how many people have approached me after I'd been visibly a-spec, or talked openly about a-spec issues, to tell me that something I'd said had helped them understand themself better.

There's a history of words being placed upon ace-spectrum people without our consent. Words like "frigid" and "hypoactive sexual desire disorder" have been used to pathologise and control people who don't love as they "should" throughout history, and most of us are keenly aware of this history. So while we might enthusiastically welcome a new person into our ranks, once they had already decided to claim a word like demi or aro for themself, we have no interest in "forcing" anyone to identify or label themself a certain way. Our community is a safe place for people who have been marginalised by compulsory sexuality and amatonormativity – the often-unquestioned assumptions that all humans are sexual beings, and that coupled, exclusive romantic love is more profound or special than other types of love. People are here because they want to be.

Out of the 160 people who filled out my initial contact form, 48 used the word "demisexual", "demiromantic" or both to describe their orientation. Of the 40 people I interviewed, 11 described themselves as demiromantic or demisexual, sometimes alongside another a-spec term like asexual, but just as often alongside an allo term like pansexual or homoromantic.

Usually defined as "forming a romantic or sexual bond only after a deep emotional connection has formed", the demi people I spoke to generally said their experiences lined up with this definition. SKW says, "To me, the term 'demisexual' refers to an individual who doesn't feel, or only rarely feels, sexual attraction to another person prior to having made a close, emotional (likely romantic) connection first." He elaborates further, saying he explains his identity by:

> highlighting the experience of having one's head turn at the sight of an attractive stranger on the street (the Distracted Boyfriend Meme being a classic depiction of this phenomenon)... a demisexual person is quite unlikely, not-unable-but-unlikely, to have these experiences.

HD, who is demiromantic and asexual, says:

> I am romantically attracted to some people if I already have a close connection and feel comfortable with them. I have felt romantic attraction to people of many genders; said attraction developed after I considered the person a friend. I have never felt any level of attraction to a stranger, and I have never felt any sexual attraction to anyone.

I myself can only think of one or two people from my past that I've experienced that intense, gut-level pull of attraction towards. A simple desire to be in their presence, to share experiences and a life with them. And in each case, this attraction only came about after we'd already been friends for quite a while.

RH, also demiromantic, says:

> I definitely know that I am romantically attracted to my partner, which only came about after we had been in a very close relationship for a while. Before that I would have described my attraction as a very close queerplatonic, in between platonic and romantic.

BC defines their experiences similarly, in terms of their past experiences with relationships:

> I usually use demisexual because I have been in a sexual relationship before (with a genderfluid trans man), but I don't seek it out or usually even have much of a libido. I use panromantic because conceptually I don't see any reason to limit who I fall in love with.

BC's comments demonstrate the complex interconnections between different orientation labels: you can be demi and pan at the same time, because one word relates to *who* you are attracted to, and the other to *when* or *how often*. One of my close friends who is demisexual also uses the word pansexual to describe themself, because while they don't experience sexual attraction until they've formed a deep emotional connection to the other person, once that connection has formed, what that person's gender is doesn't matter.

Demisexuality can also coexist alongside another ace-spectrum identity within the same person. A number of people noted that, while they could or had in the past experienced sexual attraction after an emotional bond had formed, this wasn't always the case. SS describes the way that, even if she's romantically attracted to someone, there's still no guarantee that she will feel sexual attraction:

> ...while I have had romantic interest in people across the gender spectrum, I also need to have a very well-developed and meaningful relationship with a person before any sexual interest would manifest for me, if ever. It is very rare that I would feel sexual chemistry or desire towards a person even if I do have a well-developed friendship with them. This is the language I use

> when I'm with my friends or talking about myself with people I know and trust.

SS's use of this language is context-dependent: she is an LGBTQIA+ educator as well as being a-spec, and the words she uses to describe herself change depending on the environment she's in:

> When I'm presenting in public, teaching a class, or doing advocacy work I prefer to use grey-asexual or plain asexual to describe myself. I do this because I want people to associate the word asexual with me. I want it to be very clear and present in their minds that I'm not interested in having sex, and that I don't want to talk about sex outside of a safety or educational context.

Demiromanticism especially seems to be a not very well understood identity – and I haven't seen it acknowledged at all outside the community. For EP, being demiromantic (or possibly totally aromantic – she is still figuring it out) is difficult to explain, and explaining it is work she is not willing to do with everyone. Her words echo SS, in that she's only comfortable owning the words "demiromantic" or "aromantic" with people she knows won't use them against her:

> To the uninitiated, I'd say I'm bi. Explaining it always opens up the "you just have high standards" can of worms. And maybe I do, but with the way my experience is trending, I may be entirely aromantic. And that's a bit more baggage than the average person is asking for in that moment.

Speaking more generally, I've noticed over the last few years that a surprising number of my friends and acquaintances have come out (or at least described themselves in passing) as demi, especially demisexual. I suspect that the number of people who "fit the bill" but don't have access to or want to use the language is much higher, but of course, not everyone wants or needs to claim space in the a-spec community.

Despite the fact that I (and many of my a-spec friends) have noticed that "demis are everywhere", my goal here isn't to claim "everyone's a little bit demisexual". Instead, I want to suggest that perhaps demisexuality, demiromanticism – and generally the experience of not quite fitting the conventional narrative of romantic love and sexual desire – is just much more common than we are led to believe: the conventional narrative that puts romance and sex on a pedestal to such an extent that people are afraid to admit they don't care about or don't experience certain things. It makes it difficult for the average person, a-spec or allo, to actually pinpoint how they feel about and experience sexual and romantic attraction.

Demisexuality sits on what I've come to think of as a "border" of the a-spec community. This border is an in between space, but it is also porous and lightly drawn. In my experience, demi – and it occurs to me here that the name is apt – occupies both the allo and a-spec worlds. The fact that so many people casually think of themselves as demi without being active in the larger a-spec or queer communities is further evidence that a-spec experiences are not so far removed from the "average" person's – and all of us – ace, aro, demi, grey-a – are just variations of human being.

Grey-a or greysexual

"Grey-ace", "grey-asexual" or "grey-aromantic" were the fourth most popular way the people I spoke to described themselves. Out of 160 people who filled out my contact form, 40 said they were grey-asexual, grey-aromantic or a variation on these, as well as 11 out of the 40 people I spoke to in more depth.[13]

JTS, who calls himself gay greysexual or homorromantic greysexual, says, "I usually feel aesthetic, romantic, platonic and sensual attraction. As greysexual, I hardly ever feel sexual attraction." For FG, being ace and grey-aro is simply "not feeling sexual attraction and very, very rarely feeling any desire for romantic attachment". JK, another grey-aromantic asexual, says, "I would describe it as not being interested in sexual connections or necessarily romantic connections but still wanting closeness and intimacy in a companionate and sensual matter."

There's considerable overlap between the experiences of grey-a and demi people – and grey-a is often used in a similar, or slightly less specific, way to demi. NO, who calls herself both grey-ace and demisexual, says, "I don't want sex often, and only with someone I have an emotional bond with." GH, when asked to elaborate on her a-spec identity, says:

> somewhere between grey and demi-ace, but since that's a mouthful, I'll go with a-spec. While I usually experience sexual attraction when there is a bond formed, there have been times where it hasn't been the case.

RR, who is demisexual/grey-ace says:

> I'm a sex-repulsed demi/grey-ace person, so as a concept it [sex] makes me extremely uncomfortable if that concept doesn't involve me and my partner. As an activity, it's something I've enjoyed but more so as a bonding experience than anything else.

RR's words parallel those of SS, the LGBTQIA+ educator, who says (with another pizza metaphor):

> Sex is pizza for me... My grey-asexuality means that I spend 99 per cent of my life not wanting pizza; there's a sliver of time when it sounds good, and I might choose to act on that feeling when it happens, but the everyday expectation should be that I'm not interested bordering on antipathy.

LH, who is grey-ace, says:

> I don't experience sexual attraction like allo people seem to – my emotions and romantic attractions seem very much disconnected from any sexual attraction. I find the prospect of an asexual relationship more freeing than that of a relationship with an allosexual person with regular libido and sexual expectations.

For a lot of people, including myself, "grey" is a way of creating space for uncertainty and nuance, sidestepping the need to go into too much detail, or even to fully understand or explore our own relation to sexuality and romantic attraction. LG says:

> For me, my grey aroace/aroace spec label means that while I know I don't experience sexual attraction, my romantic feelings are more nebulous. I guess the "grey" and "spec" parts are me leaving room for my feelings to change and alluding to the fact that my experiences are nuanced.

This very much tracks with my own use of the word "grey-ace": for example, I think I have felt sexual attraction before, but I'm not sure where it came from or why I felt it then and not under other circumstances. I don't know if it followed from a deepening of our relationship, or the emergence of romantic feelings, and if I'm honest, I'm not that interested in plumbing its very depths, in pinning down *exactly* what I was feeling and why.

"Grey-a", like "queer", allows one to simply say, "My feelings of romantic and sexual attraction are rare and inconsistent, nothing anyone else does or says or represents to me will necessarily produce them", and leave it at that. It allows us to express a complicated, potentially changing relationship with sexuality and romance, while not necessarily defining for anyone *else* what their exact experiences are.

Discussion questions

1. Had you heard of asexuality/ace, aromantic/aro, demi and grey-a before today? In what contexts had you encountered these words? How does this chapter's definitions match up (or not) with your previous understandings?
2. Have any of the identity terms or discussion in this chapter inspired a new way of thinking about sex, sexuality, attraction or desire?

Microlabels

This chapter and the previous one are not glossaries. I'm not here to draw neat boxes around words that, in everyday life, are more often fluid, overlapping, nebulous, contested or playful. I'm not interested in standardising terms or packaging them to make them palatable or even intelligible to outsiders. I'm only here to describe – and try to capture some of the nuance of – what I see.

At the same time, there are a number of words used by the people I spoke to, to describe their a-spec experience, that I had never heard before. Many of these words are not so much *identities* per se but instead useful descriptors, offering up an aspect of experience that might never have been articulated before. They offer space for exploration and the chance to better organise our understandings of ourselves.

Many of the terms I list below articulate aspects of my own experience that I had never been able to put into words. While I don't apply all of them to myself, absorbing their meaning has helped me think more deeply about the way I relate to sex, friendship, intimacy, romance and attraction. Lots of the people I spoke to likewise mentioned specific moments of enlightenment when they'd come across a new term that described exactly what they were experiencing. For that reason alone I think it's worth including them: perhaps some of the following words will do the same for you. (Please note this is not an exhaustive list! These are merely new-to-me terms used by the people I interviewed, or that I've come across frequently in my research.)

Aceflux

This refers to someone whose sexuality or romantic orientation fluctuates or changes over time or in different environments, while generally staying within the ace spectrum. For example, RH, who is demiromantic and aceflux, says, "I originally adopted the label aceflux when I found that my mental health condition and medication was affecting my sexual attraction and sex drive." For me, my libido – though not necessarily my feelings of attraction – fluctuates in connection with my medical transition, specifically hormone replacement therapy, so aceflux could also describe my own experience. A person's experience of fluctuating desire or attraction need not be linked to medication or even anything physical, however! Four per cent of the 2020 Ace Census respondents described themselves as "aceflux", "acefluid" or a variation thereof.

Aegosexuality

An aegosexual person is someone who may enjoy or be aroused by sexual content, masturbate or have sexual fantasies but has no desire to have sex with someone or get into a sexual relationship with another person.[1] An aegosexual person's fantasies might be in third person, "as though you're watching it on TV", and might feature fictional characters, celebrities or strangers, rather than people they know. This term was specifically coined by an a-spec person to describe an a-spec experience, in contrast to an earlier exonym, coined by psychologist Anthony Bogaert, "autochorissexual".[2] Of the Ace Census respondents, 1.3 per cent referred to themselves as some variation on "aegosexual" (a few did use the word "autochorissexual").

Allo(sexual/romantic)

This is just someone who isn't asexual or aromantic! The world allosexual/alloromantic functions similarly to "cisgender", in that it explicitly names something that had previously gone unnamed and therefore unquestioned, turning allo from an unconscious "default" into a category on equal footing with a-spec categories.

Alterous

This is a desire for emotional closeness that is not adequately described by either romantic or platonic attraction.[3] VC says, "It feels less suffocating [to use the word "alterous" than] to try and draw lines between romantic and platonic by simply acknowledging my love for friends and partners as a nonbinary type of love." Sixteen per cent of Ace Census survey respondents said they experienced alterous attraction.

Apothisexual

This is another word for sex repulsed. This describes a range of different experiences: a sex-repulsed person may be comfortable engaging with or encountering sexual content "in the wild" but not want to have sex themself, or they may be totally revolted by anything sexual whatsoever. Sex repulsion is about (sometimes visceral) physical and emotional reactions, and usually has nothing to do with a person's views on sex as a concept – all the sex-repulsed people I spoke to were sex positive from a political standpoint. Less than 1 per cent of the 2020 Ace Census respondents used this word to describe themselves.

Cupiosexual

LGBTA Wiki defines cupiosexuality as "someone who does not experience sexual attraction but still desires/likes a sexual relationship. Cupiosexuals are commonly sex-favorable but they do not have to be."[4] Put very simply, this word describes an ace-spectrum person who is not sex averse. This seems to be a relatively rare microlabel: only two people I spoke to in depth, and less than 1 per cent of the Ace Census respondents, used this term.

Limerence

Limerence is not an a-spec term; instead it is mainly used in scholarship and research on relationships more generally. This describes the intense feelings of infatuation, even obsession, that *some* people experience when entering a new (usually romantic) relationship. Limerence often has less to do with the actual object of attraction, and more to do with the limerent's idealised mental representation of that person. I don't experience (or at least I have never experienced) limerence myself, and only one of my interviewees mentioned it, but I include it here because I think it's a useful term in that it describes a concept particularly pertinent to popular culture and media portrayals of romantic and/or sexual attraction – that intense, obsessive infatuation, where you can't stop thinking about a person. The "falling" of falling in love. Intuition tells me that limerence may be a useful word if only to describe its *lack* as an aspect of a-spec experience of relationships.

Queerplatonic

This word, and related terms like queerplatonic partner, QPR or QPP, cropped up a lot as a way to describe an ideal type of relationship for many a-spec people. According to LGBTA Wiki, a QPR "bends, changes, and challenges Western culture's understanding of monogamous and committed relationships."[5] It questions the rules for telling apart romantic relationships from non-romantic relationships. It's a partnership or relationship that is committed and intimate in any number of ways, but that is not – or not quite, or not exclusively or always – romantic. RH says her experience of attraction has been "queerplatonic, in between platonic and romantic". When asked about her ideal relationship, VC says she'd like to have a queerplatonic life partner. EF says, "If I was to date, it would be more of a queerplatonic partnership situation, which would probably be with another a-spec individual." This set of terms was new to me and to a number of the people who used it. AB describes her first relationship as queerplatonic (though she didn't use the word to describe it at the time): "We were just close friends who enjoy spending time together, cuddle and occasionally kissing each other."

Like "grey-a" and "wtfromantic", queerplatonic "queers" our

understanding of how relationships should be: it's a way of sidestepping the blurry and poorly articulated border around "romance" and leaning into the fact that some intimate, committed relationships are also ambiguous, multifarious and nuanced, and that it's alright not to call something one thing or another. The word "queerplatonic" was first coined by dreamwidth users Kaz and Meloukhia/S.E. Smith in 2011.[6]

Quoi- (as in the French for "why") or wtfromantic

These terms seem to be interchangeable and represent a state of "romance confusion". Those who used them to describe themselves expressed an uncertainty, not only about their own experiences of romance and romantic attraction, but also about what romance and romantic attraction actually meant. VC sums up what being quoiromantic means to her:

> I have a complicated relationship with romance and romantic relationships. It's possible that I have experienced romantic attraction before, but I wonder if it was limerence and if other people would've perceived them differently. It's confusing for me to reflect too much on the romantic attraction, so I try to focus on the topic of romantic relationships. I don't know which behaviours and activities are romance coded beyond referring to romance-coded things in the media.

KL, who first introduced me to the word "wtfromantic", says, "I don't think I experience romantic attraction???? But I don't really know what that means??? I like being in a relationship, and my partner is sort of different from my friends but also not????" A number of people I spoke to expressed similar sentiments

– confusion around the precise nature of romance vs other types of feelings – without necessarily naming it in this way. Around thirteen per cent of the Ace Census respondents used quoi- or wtfromantic to describe themselves.

Discussion questions

1. Did any of the "microlabels" in this chapter resonate with you or your experiences? If so, how does it make you feel to know there are words for what you've experienced?
2. How many of the "microlabel" words did you know already? How many had you heard before but didn't know what they meant? How many were completely new?
3. Aside from their basic definitions, have any of the microlabel words in this chapter inspired any new way of thinking about sex, sexuality, attraction or desire?
4. Take two of these identity terms and look them up online. Try to find a definition for each one from someone who uses the word to describe themself. Observe how the meanings of these words can fluctuate based on who is using it.

When Language Isn't Enough

Note: This chapter contains a brief mention of sexual violence.

As much as I love language, there are things it can't do and times when it fails. As much as I like having the words to express myself, sometimes even "nonbinary" – a word I've been using to describe myself for years, a word that's literally on the front cover of my first book – feels like it's too much, bogged down by all the expectations and assumptions people make when they hear it. It feels freer to let my gender remain unnamed, un-dissected – to let it just exist.

The history of words, and the contexts around them, can have just as much of an effect on how they are used as their definitions. When it comes to language, my travels in the community have revealed two different attitudes towards microlabels like the ones I discussed in the last chapter. Many of us embrace terms like aceflux, alterous attraction and grey-aromantic, not necessarily because there are specific aceflux or grey-aro communities we want to be part of, but because these words accurately and precisely express ways of being that, for most of human history, have had no expression. In order to explore and celebrate something, it must be first allowed to exist. In order for it to exist in my mind and yours – for its existence to be shared between us – it must first be named.

But at the same time, many of us, for example those who just use "ace" to describe their orientation and leave it at that, feel uneasy with labelling something that may be too slippery or changeable to truly pin down, or that we might not be comfortable sharing in detail with the rest of the world. I personally feel that, even if there was one single, very long word that expressed exactly my experience of sexuality and attraction, I wouldn't use it to describe myself. For one thing, I have doubts as to whether, deep down, I even *have* an essential or inherent sexuality or set orientation. Like my gender, I want to *live* my experience, not describe it.

I also don't think the word would be very useful. For one thing, if I'm the only one who knows what it means, what's the point? For another, I don't just use words to describe myself, I also use them to declare membership in a certain group. When I call myself "ace", I'm describing my sexuality, but I'm also expressing solidarity with the other people who use that word. What "ace" precisely means to my lived experience is less important than the fact that, in using it, I share it with others. The same goes for "queer" and "trans" – these are words I use to describe myself a *lot*, but like "ace" they lack a set definition. These words ask more questions than they answer, but that's not a bad thing, because they do what they need to: align me visibly with the queer, trans and a-spec communities. Asking the questions these words allow me to ask is an essential part of my work as an activist.

For many, our use of language has to do with a very human desire to *belong* somewhere, to feel like part of a lineage and larger community of other people like ourselves, to take a place among them and share their struggle for social transformation.

There are any number of words I could use to more accurately describe my lived experience – AFAB nonbinary, grey-asexual, quoi- or wtfromantic – but "queer" and "trans", "ace" and "a-spec" are the words I claim for myself.

For many of us, that signal of group membership is the only thing that needs to be put into words – the rest can remain unarticulated. LG, who just uses "aroace", "grey aroace" or "aroace spec", said:

> I usually don't like using more specific a-spec terms because I find them limiting. My asexuality and aromanticism manifest in many different ways and I don't feel like adding secondary or hyper-specific terms to it. In fact, the only reason I tend to add the "bi" bit in front of it is because I want to reinforce that spectrum bit. It took me a long time to come to terms with the fact that romantic attraction can be an ill-defined grey area for me. I can feel completely aromantic most of the time but then occasionally crave a romantic relationship or develop a crush.

For LG, specificity of language is not only limiting but maybe impossible: their experience of attraction is changeable and ill-defined, and trying to pin it down with more specific terms isn't helpful.

For others, the accuracy of the words we use is less important than how they can be used in different contexts. SS, who identifies most closely with demisexual but uses grey-asexual or just asexual to describe herself to others, recounted the way people have treated her differently, depending on their understandings of the words she uses:

> In the past when I used demisexual to describe myself to others, I found that my boundaries weren't taken as seriously when

> I expressed them. My use of demi resulted in an assumption that, "Okay we're friends now, so you'll find me sexually attractive." And when I pushed back and refused flirtation or sexual contact, people became unpleasant (and a few times they were violent). Using demi made people think they had a chance of a sexual encounter with me if they just waited long enough. Once I switched to using grey-asexual in public spaces and when meeting new people, I found that my boundaries were more readily respected, and I overall received less push-back and more support from those around me. Having the word "asexual" within my identity produces the result I want.

For SS, her choice of identity label was a matter of safety. Because people were prone to mistaking her use of the word demisexual for a tacit admission that she would automatically find them sexually attractive once they had been friends for "long enough", SS was forced to change her use of language to protect herself, regardless of whether it described her experience.

I, and lots of people I spoke to, also expressed a specific worry around detailed language, used just for the sake of taxonomic accuracy. KL summed it up neatly when explaining why they used "ace" instead of "asexual": "Ace...feels more casual and less clinical."

By writing this book, I don't want to give the impression that my definitions are the only ones, or that I "own" my community's language. That language has been created on purpose to be unresolved and not owned by any one person.

That's why I take pains to say that these chapters are not glossaries; trying to pin down a microlabel with a precise definition fails to capture the spirit of these words, but it's also potentially dangerous.

Because it also depends on who is using the words. There's a long history, in the West at least, where the person who writes something down owns it, from monks dropping Christian themes and values into pagan tales[1] to the doctors who turned asexuality into a disease by giving it an entry in the diagnostic manual. *Technically accurate* words have been applied to my community by outsiders, with the intention of categorising and fixing us, rather than allowing asexuality to simply be an essential part of who we are. Terms such as "hypoactive sexual desire disorder" have been, and still are, used by medical professionals to take away our sexual and bodily agency. In these cases, words have caused real harm.

Seen in this light, the stakes surrounding me writing this book seem somewhat higher. It has become accepted practice, for writers from both inside and outside the queer community, to write "explainers" of various parts of that community – dictionaries in which new-fangled language around gender and sexuality are unpacked and repackaged for the consumption of the reader. My own first book somewhat fits that model, though I did my best to allow for the messiness and nuance of identity.

But knowing the complex history, in which my identity – asexual – has been turned into a dictionary entry, and in which people like me have been displayed on TV to entertain an audience, I've become wary of dictionaries and what they represent. I can't help but draw a parallel in my mind between a dictionary – in which each subcategory of a-spec experience is pinned down, neatly bounded by a concise definition – and a display case, a cabinet of curiosities, where I and everyone in my community are arranged for the delectation of an allo public. I can't in good conscience allow this book to fall into that mould.

Over and over while writing, I've had to think about my own place at the intersection of observer and observed. I've questioned my own role in writing a book that offers up my community to the public eye. I've questioned my own instincts and research methods and thought processes, which for better or for worse are shaped by my academic and scientific training. I've second-guessed everything from my use of questionnaires and statistics to my decision to try to provide definitions at all.

The community itself is keenly aware of the difference between labels that we have claimed for ourselves and labels that have been put on us without our consent: just look at the creation of "aegosexual" in response to "autochorissexual". In these cases, we must ask ourselves what, and who, words are for. My experience of attraction and sexuality is private, and most of us are not comfortable with being, as the authors of *Asexualities: Feminist and Queer Perspectives* put it, "objects of scholarly scrutiny".[2]

I have no doubt that writing the explainer would have been easier. It's easier to create methodical, clear-cut categories, to say "these people are asexual and here's what that means", without ambiguity or context. But this approach doesn't exist in a vacuum, and I don't have the luxury of scientific distance. No one writing about my community, aware of its history, should have that luxury. Instead, I've tried to seek nuance, to allow uncertainty to flourish, even to celebrate it. In the face of so much pressure to explain ourselves, pressure to be certain, the ease with which so many a-spec people hold onto the ambiguity, blurriness and changeability of human experience is both a strength and a radical act.

Bringing experiences like "aromantic" and "aegosexual" into the English language is to declare that there is space for the people they describe. In creating language to use amongst ourselves we aren't "making up labels"; instead, we're trying to create space where interstitial, undefined, transitory or fluid aspects of our experience can be allowed to exist.

But at the same time, the power of our language lies in the way it is constantly and collaboratively growing and changing.

To put something down on paper is to lend it permanence and rigidity, and by definition this fails to capture its fluidity. With each step the a-spec community takes into the light of visibility and mainstream acceptance, we will have to continually navigate this tension.

Perhaps ironically, both the impulses I describe above – the development of neologisms to declare and even celebrate a marginalised set of experiences, and the rejection of precise taxonomic language – feel very a-spec to me. Our community is characterised by a radical and nuanced use of language, carving out spaces that have until now been marginal or non-existent, but also by a comfort with ambiguity. There is power in naming yourself, but there is also power in being unnameable.

Discussion questions

1. What kind of words do you use to describe yourself? These don't have to be sexuality labels, but could refer to other aspects of your personal identity, marginalised or not – Scottish, Black, midwesterner, gamer, East London, Hearts or Hibs supporter. Take some time to think about the words you use to describe yourself to others.
2. What are these labels useful for? What do they allow you to do? What are some of their limitations?
3. What are the different contexts in which you call yourself one thing or another? For example, when I'm among writer friends, I'm a writer. But when I'm explaining my work to non-writers, I'm an "author". See if you can identify where this pressure to change your use of language comes from.

Coming (and Being) Out

As a person belonging to a number of different queer identities, I've come out a few times in my life, with varying levels of drama. I've run the gamut from tearful car rides and baffled, frustrating, confrontational conversations to complete non-events, where the person I'm coming out to just says, "Oh, I thought so."

The first time I came out as ace, in the conventional sense, was to my now ex-partner. We had just started going out, and they were the first person I'd dated since discovering – or more accurately accepting – that I was ace, and at the time I wasn't yet comfortable with that fact.

I remember agonising for an hour over what was by all accounts a fairly short text message. After hitting "send" I threw my phone in a drawer and went for a long walk. I wasn't sure what I was afraid would happen, but I knew I dreaded reading the response. This was the first time I had put what I'd long known about myself into words, and what's more actually *told* someone else.

It was intensely difficult, and thinking back on it now I think I'd have been happy to *never* have to say it out loud. I had a strong sense at the time that I was only doing so because I assumed it would cause problems further down the line for our relationship, maybe even kill it in the cradle.

The response I'd been dreading, the confirmation that my disinterest in sex meant we'd never work as a couple, and that by extension I'd never work as a couple with *anyone*, didn't come.

Instead, my partner answered my disclosure with one of their own: that they were demisexual and also had little interest in sex.

Compared to some other coming-outs in my life, this conversation went as well as could have been expected, ending with a shared disclosure that I'm sure brought the two of us closer together. Our relationship lasted years and when we eventually broke up, our sexualities had nothing to do with it.

As I've said, this was the only time I've "officially" come out as ace to someone. Unlike my nonbinary trans gender, which is pretty much obvious to anyone who looks at me – and which means that any conversation with a new person involves a "coming out" of sorts – my a-spec identity is mostly invisible. Unlike conversations about pronouns, dress codes or formal titles, it simply does not come up in everyday conversation, meaning that outside of a relationship context, it hardly ever needs disclosure.

This is a double-edged sword: in most contexts, a-spec people can "pass" for allo, for whatever nebulous benefit that might confer. But it also means that it's that much harder to be visible to each other; an a-spec person can't take part in the community if they're not "out" in at least some capacity. Coming out and visibility go hand in hand, and because visibility is so complicated for a-spec people, coming out is too.

There's something of a cultural narrative in the West – of a person "coming out of the closet" once, globally, and thereafter living their truth for all to see – but that narrative doesn't work for most a-spec people. Because we are often invisible, and people tend not to readily believe in things they can't see, for a-spec people it's not always as simple as saying "I am aromantic" or "I am demisexual" and leaving it at that: the reality is often much messier.

Before an a-spec person can come out to anyone else, they must first come out to themself, and visibility, being able to see yourself reflected in the community, is essential for that. Near the beginning of this book I mentioned how Yasmin Benoit, one of the most visible members of the aroace community right now, experienced a lag between "discovering" asexuality and choosing to claim that word for herself. Before she was able to "[meet] other asexual people really, enough to kind of gauge like, what the community was actually like",[1] it seemed like there was nothing there for her.

A number of people I spoke to echoed this experience. Many recalled that, while discovering the language of asexuality and the existence of the community was essential for them to be able to claim that language and space for themselves, that claiming didn't always happen immediately – whether, like Benoit, because they didn't see people who resembled themselves in those spaces, or because vestigial insecurity and internalised aphobia meant that they weren't yet comfortable enough with themselves to embrace being a-spec.

For me, the latter was very much the case: I've had the words for a long time, but becoming comfortable in my a-spec identity was, and still is, an ongoing process. Before I could come out to anyone else, I had to fully believe both that I was asexual – or at least on the ace spectrum – and also, crucially, that I lived in a world where this might truly be okay. Even today, I'm still sometimes uncomfortable discussing my own relationship to the aromantic constellation of identities, because I'm not sure if I belong there or not. As a result, I don't often talk about that side of me.

The narrowness of ace and a-spec representation surely plays a part as well: even among the ace community, I rarely see people who are visibly okay on their own. The pressure from outside the community to present ourselves as "normal in every other way" means that lots of ace representation centres around aces getting into otherwise-normative couple relationships. It's only recently, with the new visibility of queerplatonic and anarchic relationships, that I've seen models of relationship that I felt I could embody.

Once you've embraced your own a-spec identity, if you've been raised in a culture (US-American, for example as I was) that normalises and places huge social value on the romantic-sexual nuclear family, asserting that part of yourself to others becomes more than a simple disclosure: it can become a battle to convince people that you exist. How do you prove a negative – especially when everyone around you is telling you "You just haven't found the right person yet" or "How will you know unless you try it?"

When you come out as a-spec to an allo person, especially someone like a family member who has a personal stake in your continued participation in compulsory sexuality, it's easy for them to simply refuse to believe you. They can try to convince you that you don't know yourself, or choose to pretend the conversation never happened. And because living as "openly" a-spec is not visible in the same way as starting to date someone of the same gender as you, or changing your gender presentation, many of us remain invisible *even after* coming out to the people close to us. For these people, this "coming out" happens over and over; it will be a continuing process for as long as the communities and environments we live in maintain that allo default.

As I mentioned in the chapter on friendships and family relationships, coming out as a-spec becomes, for many of us, a moment when others prioritise their own needs over ours. Coming out to parents and older relatives, many of the people

I spoke to found that the conversation had been conveniently forgotten the next time questions of marriage or starting a family came up; if they were acknowledged at all, aromanticism or asexuality were treated by older relatives as immaterial, "just words", compared to the very real obligations of having children and continuing the family line. As HD says:

> I have come out to my parents multiple times as asexual. The first time they told me I would grow out of it. Each of them shortly after gave me speeches about how the media was oversexualised and what was portrayed on TV about attraction and relationships was not realistic. I don't entirely know if my parents remember I identify as asexual, we don't bring it up, I feel disinclined to after their three or four initial reactions.

When asked if there were contexts in which she had to hide her asexuality, HBJ said, "possibly around my parents and extended family...their assumption that the whole world is straight unless obviously otherwise means it doesn't come up very often. There was more pressure to talk about when I was going to provide grandchildren than there was to talk about my orientation." HBJ went on to say that she would probably never come out as a-spec to her parents: "Some battles aren't worth fighting. I know myself and I'm comfortable with my orientation, and that's sufficient for me." FG, when asked if her family knew she was ace and grey-aro, said:

> My family don't know, and I plan to take this to my grave. My family is very conservative, the only person who isn't openly homophobic is my mother, and even then she's biased against every other LGBTQIA+ identity and thinks they're "made up". I never want to come out to them. This means having to play

> straight for a lot of interactions, which is probably less stressful than the risks of being out to them.

A number of people also mentioned how a lack of access to language, which prevents allos from understanding what asexuality or aromanticism actually are, further complicated their coming out process. BC says:

> My family doesn't know. I've given up talking to them about my queerness – they're Catholics who would prefer that I stay in an easily comprehensible box like "gay" that they can safely ignore. There's a lot we just don't talk about.

CD says, "My parents still hope for grandchildren from me, but I see no difference in outcome between their assuming me to be a heterosexual woman with PTSD (which I do have), and my being an asexual woman."

These experiences, of rejection coupled with a lack of understanding, aren't unique to a-spec people; while working on my first book, about nonbinary gender, I regularly encountered people whose families had simply not made an effort to understand. Rather than something interesting or unique to be celebrated, part of what makes them who they are, many family members saw an interviewee's nonbinary gender as something "weird" that interfered with their own expectations of that person. In so many instances, a parent's personal investment in the system of binary gender was prioritised over the wellbeing of their child.

From an outside perspective, it may seem easiest and most empowering for an a-spec person not to bother coming out at all to family, instead simply stepping away, disavowing blood family and – as many of us do – establishing chosen family and friendship support networks instead.[2] But for many a-spec people, the reality is not so simple.

During the Q&A portion of the event, one audience member of the 2021 AceCon East- and Southeast Asian Aces panel said, "People who say you should just 'cut your family off' if they aren't accepting don't seem to really experience family in the same way as me. Have you ever been told that?" Jules, a panelist from Vietnam, had this to say:

> I have heard this so many times in my life. Especially in this generation [Gen Z] the problem is when Gen Y...have been under the pressure of having to commit to their family, because their parents are directly coming out from the war (in this context the Vietnam war, 1955 to 1975). They're born 80s, 90s, and they now have the responsibility to take care of their parents. Because Vietnam had a very difficult period in the 80s. We struggled to find food, jobs, to provide for our kids, to find adequate education. So it became like a burden for Gen Y to come back to their family. Because of that, they tell us, Gen Z, "You should just go. You should leave. Because I have been here and they are not listening to me, they are not accepting my sexuality, the best chance for you is to just go." And I think the people in that situation, they've been through so much that they have to say this.
>
> But on the other hand, the older generation, they have so much problem [sic] on their own. You pass down survival kits to your children. They tell the kids what they know. They want them to be hetero, so they can get a more smooth way in life. That's how they view it. So to change their perspective, from that point, is so difficult. I just think that, for our parents to not understand our sexuality, but to accept it, is a tough task. Because everything they have is coming from their experience.

> So we have to come out, not just to show ourselves that we exist, but to help our parents know the world better.
>
> I have heard some stories that our parents are asexual, but they have struggled so much that they have that guilt for their life. And maybe if we come out, help some of them to realise, "Oh, they're asexual and they're proud of that... They are just them." Then we can have conversations with equal sides, where both respect each other.
>
> So to cut your family off is not exactly okay, because if you get through that barrier, you get to know your parents better... Parents give us life, we are not a burden to them. We are a gift that they have inherited from the sky. If you are a child, and you are looking at your parents and see all their struggles, you don't leave them.

While younger Western queers are encouraged, especially online, to cut ties completely with anyone who doesn't accept them for who they are, this approach to coming out and being open about our identities fails to extend empathy to the people we're coming out to, or allow them the possibility of coming to understand.

Jules' is an example of a perspective often overlooked in Western, English-language discussions of a-spec identities, namely perspectives acknowledging that experiences of living within amatonormativity are not the same all over the world. Non-Western a-spec perspectives complexify our picture of the ways that history and politics have shaped romantic and sexual norms – and a handful of these perspectives I will explore in the section on "Cultural background and racialisation". Often, these are ignored in favour of "party lines", the mainstream narratives that allow us to present a unified front as a community. But it is *because* the language and political movement of asexuality has mostly been articulated by people from Western and

Anglophone countries – often countries that were themselves perpetrators of colonialism or imperialism – that it's important for us to listen to the perspectives of a-spec people from outside the Anglophone world.

An exclusively Western perspective fails to take into account the mitigating context of culture and history: in this case, the effects of intergenerational trauma on our ideas about sexuality. For older people who have lived through war or colonialism, understanding the nuances of asexuality or aromanticism may be a hard task, in a different way than they are a hard task for an American or British older person to understand. Considering that a-spec identities are so often articulated only in English, it's not hard to see how they might even be perceived as Western imports. In these cases, when coming out, the most productive or responsible thing to do might not be to cut off one's family, but to be mindful of where they are coming from, and to trust in their capacity to learn and grow.

Aside from family pressures, many people mentioned other external obstacles that had conspired to prevent them from coming out as a-spec. IJ sums up these difficulties and how they've been shaped by our current cultural moment which, while it has gifted us with new vocabulary to talk about our experiences, has also opened the door for outsiders to express their opinions, speak over us or make assumptions about what it's like to be us:

> I find it very difficult to talk about it [being a-spec] with others, particularly due to my lack of words and not being comfortable really discussing it most of the time. I also often assume that they won't understand and have also spent a lot of time on the internet seeing various arguments around a-spec identities, which puts me off talking to friends who would probably be at least vaguely supportive for fear they will say something

> disparaging, or be thinking something negative. The internet discourse over the past number of years around asexuality and its validity as an identity...is a major reason that I have issues talking about it and feeling like it is something I can be open about, as I worry it'll make people think of me badly or assume things about me that aren't true.

The proliferation of new ways to talk about gender and sexuality has also seen the crystallisation of a reactionary movement, perceiving a (quite real) threat to the status quo. The idea that something previously (though not always!) thought to be biologically essential, hardwired and universal might actually be fluid or socially constituted – that the hierarchies our society rests upon might in fact be made of sand – can inspire fear and confusion, which in turn can inspire exclusionary politics that can put a-spec people, indeed all LGBTQ+ people, in danger.

Online (at least in the UK) this reactionary politics is most visibly popular with TERFs, or trans-exclusionary radical feminists, many of whom are vocally uncomfortable with the kind of fluidity and egalitarian use of language that is common in both the a-spec and trans communities. My interviewees themselves were aware of this connection: JH mentioned the "preponderance of TERFs" in today's discussions of gender/sexuality, and BC described disclosing their a-spec identity to new friends as "a good way to pick out the TERFs".

This reaction to change has led to a concept of "snowflake" culture, the idea that the (usually young) people embracing queer ideas of sexual and gender fluidity are somehow doing it for attention or social clout, and that the subversive, egalitarian language they're using to articulate their experiences – because that language doesn't belong to the officially sanctioned vocabulary of binary sex/gender – is actually meaningless.

A-spec exists at an interstice of complicated facets of identity; it's compatible (or even, as I'll explore later in this chapter, correlates) with all sorts of other non-normative experiences of gender and sexuality. So, many of us have to contend with the tension between a dynamic, fluid way of being that resists being put into words, and very real social pressure to put it into words regardless, in order for it to exist in the minds of others. As such, the stereotype of the "special snowflake" has been weaponised against many people in the a-spec community and used to dismiss or silence us.

The environment of hostility created by TERFs and "gender-critical" ideologues has led many of us to feel trepidation around publicly identifying as "more than one thing", as if identity labels were gaudy parade medals and not a simple attempt to put words to feelings. A number of the people I spoke to said they were reluctant to be seen "changing their mind", for example switching from calling themselves "gay", when they realised they weren't attracted to the opposite sex, to "ace", upon realising they weren't attracted to anyone – even though the less-accurate term "gay" was *always* going to be available to them first.

Because of this pressure, many people recalled self-policing, managing their coming out in such a way that it was more palatable to others, or just not coming out at all. For example, when asked where pressure to hide her grey-asexuality comes from, LH said:

> Allonormativity, and actually also heteronormativity: it feels like I've already come out as non-straight, so adding asexuality on top feels very special-snowflakey when surrounded by cishet allo people. If people didn't assume that I'm a straight allosexual woman, it wouldn't be so damn obnoxious having to correct all of their assumptions.

RH, who is demiromantic, quoiromantic and aceflux, echoed LH, saying:

> I worry about being judged for having a very specific identity, or one that would need explaining, and being viewed as a "snowflake". I also don't want to repeat my past experiences of aphobic and biphobic arguments online and offline, from people who want to remove ace and aro from the LGBT+ umbrella...and [who] disagree with people using the split-attraction model to describe themselves. I still feel a certain level of shame because of society and media's idea of what people who have sex without romance are like, as well as well-meaning friends who didn't understand my experience, and so said insensitive things.

But a number of the people I spoke to had the experience of "trying on" multiple identities before settling on their current one, for any number of reasons, depending on the environment or community one lives in, or the fact that identity can and does change, despite the "born this way" narrative popular in mainstream LGBT+ discourse. In this way, articulating one's identity is like learning a new language: when you're desperate to communicate, you use the words available to you, even if they're not the best ones. As you learn more, you're able to use better ones. It's not a matter of changing your mind as much as getting to know yourself better, learning the "language" of what makes you who you are.

EF eloquently explains the messiness of identity and the insecurities it can rake up, and why it's so important to be patient and lenient with yourself through the coming out process, as long and circuitous as it might be:

> As I mentioned earlier, I identified as a lesbian when I realised

> that aroace fit me so much more. For me, it was very difficult. I felt like a complete fraud to go from identifying as gay to identifying as ace, as though I'd been lying to everyone, that I'd gone through a "phase". I was scared that nobody was going to believe that I was really aroace because I'd already come out as gay, and bi before that – and some people didn't! Also I'd come out four times (including my enby identity) at this point – I was tired of not knowing myself and was scared that I'd never get there and just be constantly stuck in a permanent identity crisis. Of course through doing some personal development I know now that the whole "coming out" process is totally different for everyone, and that a label is used to describe how you feel at that moment. I honestly felt like I was a lesbian, but that was before I truly understood how I experienced sexual and romantic attraction.

When asked if the people they'd come out to had been accepting of their identity, EF said:

> Generally I would say yes, but in general I've had to do a lot of explaining/clearing up of misconceptions about asexuality/aromanticism with even my best friends – i.e. it not being a choice/that I can still *actually* have sex/that the fact I'm not a virgin doesn't take away from being asexual/that a QPR is not just having a best friend. One friend who I came out to said that I love to attach labels onto myself, and, because my relationships were quite often pretty toxic, that I hadn't found the right person yet. Another friend said that I was only identifying as aroace to look special, and that I'd be "straight with a boyfriend" in five years – like even if I did have a "boyfriend", I would still be aroace!

All of us, allo, ace, gay, straight, are always in process, always figuring stuff out, and changing the language we use, or even changing our minds, is not the end of the world. While it might seem to allo people that we're being flighty or attention-seeking, you can be sure that none of us are coming out lightly. We've all already questioned, censored and policed ourselves at length. As RR says, "Accept that it's my choice to label myself and there aren't 'too many' labels nor any that are 'unnecessary'." Or as EP puts it, "If I don't have answers, that doesn't mean I'm wrong."

Discussion questions

1. Have you had to "come out" to anyone in your life? How easy or complicated was the process?
2. What would have made the process easier?
3. If you've come out multiple times or as multiple identities, think about your experiences of coming out. How did they differ and why?

A-spec and the LGBTQ+ Community

I'm queer. And because I'm writing it, this book is a queer book. I've been going to Pride marches since I was in my teens, and I wore a suit to my high school prom, even before I knew what "trans" meant. For as long as I've had a concept of "sexual orientation", even if I didn't quite know what that orientation *was*, I have never thought of myself as "straight".

I bring this up because my asexual and grey-aromantic identity is not a gap, an unticked box, something missing from my orientation. Instead, it's a fundamental part of my queerness, a constitutive part of what makes me queer, as much as my nonbinary, trans gender. For most of my life, queer spaces[1] are those in which I've learned about and been able to express myself most truly.

I was somewhat surprised to find that the vast majority of the people I spoke to told me they considered themselves queer or part of the LGBT(QIA+) community, by virtue of being ace, aro, demi or grey-a. I wasn't surprised because I didn't think we belonged, but because – as I'll explore later on in the chapter – we are generally invisible, even or especially within the queer community. Even if they hadn't, the very preponderance of people I spoke to who described themselves as queer *and*, gay *and*, trans *and* a-spec shows us that the queer and a-spec communities are very closely intertwined indeed.

The strongest overarching impression I got of my interviewees' own relationships with, and experiences moving within, the LGBTQ+ community was that, while some people had not personally felt welcome or comfortable there, no one thought that a-spec people *were not* or *could not be* part of it.

Looking at the 160 people who answered my Google form to register interest in the book, even without looking at the a-spec specific labels, there's a cornucopia of terms for describing sexuality, romantic orientation and ways of experiencing love and attraction: queer, pansexual, lesbian, homoromantic, gay-oriented, panromantic, bisexual, demibisexual, biromantic, panplatonic seeking queerplatonic relationships.

A huge number of people, nearly 20 per cent, also selected the option "not entirely sure/figuring out" in the "orientation" field. In contrast, only 3 of the 160 described themselves as "heteroromantic", and not one person described themself as "straight" or "heterosexual".

Out of the people I spoke to in more depth, over half described themselves as "queer", as well as or in place of a more specific word like "demisexual" or "panromantic". Like the people who preferred "ace" or "a-spec" over a more specific word, lots of people said that "queer" felt more comfortable for them than more specific labels. A number also said that, outside the a-spec community (where people might not know what "demisexual" or "quoiromantic" means, or who might be less receptive to the idea of an a-spec identity than to a more widely understood LGBTQ+ label), they would default to "queer" when asked about their orientation.

"Queer" is a very useful word here: for someone whose experience of attraction, desire and sexuality might be ambiguous, undecided, in progress or wilfully un-articulated, "queer" offers a huge amount of space to play around in. It offers a way of articulating our experience without – as IJ described it – "dissecting it".

This sense of kinship with specifically *queer* experience isn't a coincidence: over and over it struck me, while looking at the words of my interviewees, that the categories of sexuality, romantic orientation and even gender are not sharp or discrete but rather porous. There was huge overlap and bleed between the different ways in which one could "be" queer, and the people who shared their experiences with me were themselves aware of this: as CF puts it, "there is an intersectional character to many a-spec people that deepens the connection between the two communities".

A great many of the people I spoke to – and I myself – were only able to find out they were a-spec in the first place *because* of the LGBTQ+ community, having gained access to the language of the ace spectrum in a larger context of LGBTQ+ identities and sexual diversity education.

Conventional sex education takes as a given that pupils will both want sex *and* form heterosexual couples – these two behaviours go hand in hand in the world of sex ed (and heteronormativity), and deviation from this norm in *any way* is rarely acknowledged. This alone creates a basic commonality of experience between any young person whose sexuality and experience of desire and attraction do not match up with that of their peers or what the adults in their life expect from them. For many people, this sense of alienation or outsiderhood extends beyond adolescence, and leads to an abiding and inextricable intertwining between a-spec identity and a wider sense of *queerness*.

Realising we are aro or demi or ace may be the first time in our lives that many of us come into conflict with the sexual status quo, the first time we fail or refuse to conform to normative expectations and start thinking of ourselves as *different*.

With that understanding comes an awareness of the fragility of the roles we're made to play. In the same way that a person's ambivalence about their gender might go hand in hand with an ambivalence about sex and sexual performance, all these different facets of queerness are so tightly tied to one another in the ways we are taught to construct identity, that it's easy to see how taking that first step away from the norm, snipping one thread, might cause the whole thing to unravel.

Apart from the odd joke from my high-school peers about reproduction by budding, I myself had never heard the word asexuality until I entered what would become my first queer space, Tumblr, in the early 2010s. I first used the site when I was in my late teens, and it was here that I first encountered the idea of aromanticism and asexuality as legitimate orientations in their own right, alongside a wider array of non-normative genders and sexualities. (I first heard the word "nonbinary" in this community as well.) Queer spaces and the LGBTQ+ community were fundamental to my "discovery" of asexuality. For me, at that time, the a-spec and LGBTQ+ communities were functionally one and the same.

The importance of the LGBTQ+ community – its vocabulary and its elders – as a bank of knowledge and history for a-specs first coming into their own, then, cannot be understated. For many of us, learning about queerness is our first hint that there is more than meets the eye when it comes to sexuality and desire, and that there are possibilities beyond what is demanded of us by society. As LH puts it, "I think most a-spec people consider themselves LGBT+. At least the ones I know... And they often started, like me, by just feeling non-straight, zeroing in on asexuality later."

Because of this close connection, many of the people who shared their experiences with me also explicitly said they felt more comfortable discussing a-spec issues with other LGBTQ+ people and felt a sense of commonality across specific identity boundaries. LG, for example, said:

> Honestly I don't care about interacting with other a-spec people specifically as much as it's important to me that I interact with queer people in general (and I do include a-spec people when I say queer people). My experiences can sometimes be intersectional between identities and even if someone is allo, our experiences can be very similar. For example I have a friend who is bi and allo and their experience with trying to conform to heterosexuality and dating a straight dude is similar to my experience pressuring myself to be allo and date a guy I was not attracted to in any way, shape or form.

SKW, too, says that he was first able to articulate his demisexuality with the help of his nonbinary, pansexual romantic partner, who was already used to moving within inclusive queer spaces. SKW says of his partner, "they have been very instrumental in having me question and explore some of these aspects of my own identity; things that otherwise had been taken for granted, or just not truly thought about".

A-spec people have always, in some form, existed, even if the words we used to describe ourselves were different or non-existent, and asexuality has been counted alongside or as part of the bi+ umbrella, as another group whose sexualities were "neither one nor the other".[2]

AB, one of the first people I spoke to when I started writing this book, said, when asked whether the LGBTQ+ and a-spec communities were connected:

> Yes, some LGBTQ communities talk about asexuality (at least

> those who actively try to be inclusive and not only focus on mlm and wlw issues). It's important to note that a-spec people used to be part of the bisexual community since its beginning (the bi label included any person that was "neither straight nor gay" and actively included asexuals who then would go by both labels in the 1960s). In that instance, bi history is a-spec history. And queer communities are and will always be a-spec communities.

In 1907 in New Orleans, pastor Carl Schlegel was documented as advocating for equality under law for gay, straight, bi *and* ace people: "Let the same laws for all the intermediate stages of sexual life: the homosexuals, heterosexuals, bisexuals, asexuals, be legal as they are now in existence for the heterosexuals."[3] In the 1950s, the transgender magazine *Transvestia* published a series of articles on what they called "a-sexuality"[4] – not to mention the Barnard College activists with the "choose your own label" sign.[5]

This knowledge is relatively common within the a-spec community – with grassroots researchers such as Tumblr users Autismserenity and Lee from Aceing History scouring the archives to bring to light a semblance of queer a-spec history – but it's not very well known outside of it, and the notion that "asexuality didn't exist until the nineties" is a common refrain used by people trying to invalidate our identities.

But if you look at the facts, we face discrimination,[6] dehumanisation and pathologisation, all of which will sound familiar to anyone with basic knowledge of the gay rights movement; it's clear that a-spec and LGBQ communities share experiences of being an oppressed minority orientation, even if the challenges that individual identities face aren't precisely the same.

And even if we set aside the criteria of shared struggle, with many questioning if "suffering" and "oppression" should be the basis on which we decide entry to these communities[7] – there is still a lot to unite them. Neither has a strict boundary; their borders are in fact often contested – as the tension I explore later in this chapter demonstrates. As CD puts it, the communities "are connected by their presence outside of what my society considers 'traditional' relationships, and by their common experience and understanding that there is no single way for two people to love each other".

But despite this long and intertwined history, and my instinctual understanding since I was a child that my (a)sexuality and (a)romanticism were part of what made me queer, I haven't always felt comfortable in my a-spec identity within queer spaces. There have been times when I've moved in those spaces and felt like my asexuality alienated me, sometimes even more than in straight contexts.

I remember a Pride march in my city, a good few years ago. I'd spent the day marching and hanging out with a group of fellow trans people, and we'd all gone back to someone's flat to rest. None of us knew each other very well and so in the absence of common ground, the conversation turned to kink and sexual preference.

I let myself recede into the background. I was not yet out as ace, even fully to myself, though I certainly knew the conversation was making me uncomfortable – and I felt guilty for feeling uncomfortable. I was already socially exhausted from a day of hanging out with strangers, and I didn't have the energy to deal with the stares, the dismissal or the overbearing apologies I'd come to expect whenever I (seldom) disclosed my identity. But I also didn't have the energy to sit through a conversation I knew I would be utterly excluded from.

As I was trying to think of a polite way to excuse myself and go home, one of the other people in the room asked if everyone present was comfortable talking about sex. This question, essentially, amounted to that person seeking consent from the group;

it wasn't standard practice in the spaces I moved in, and to this day I still appreciate that person asking.

But as I felt the eyes of the room drift towards me, I clammed up. As much as I didn't want to sit through a long and graphic conversation about other people fucking each other, the idea of outing myself to the whole room, the prospect of having to explain myself and have everyone walk on eggshells around me for the rest of the evening, was even worse. I assumed I was the only a-spec person there (even though I probably wasn't) and the idea of being singled out because of it made me deeply uncomfortable.

While if this happened today I might have been more comfortable speaking up, at the time I simply excused myself, leaving behind a queer space that, up until then, had been a safe and welcoming one. It was a very disillusioning moment, and it took me a long time to understand both why it made me feel this way and where the obligatory sex positivity that had so alienated me came from.

Even despite the fact that so many of us already occupy queer spaces in other capacities – that so many of us are a-spec *and* another queer identity – there is tension around the idea of our taking up space within the LGBTQ+ community in our own right as ace, aro, demi or grey-a. This means our experiences of moving within LGBTQ+ spaces can be uneasy or fraught.

SKW, for instance, mentioned that, "the queer community has a tendency to ignore a-spec people, or to be dismissive of how especially the behaviour of allo members might impact a-spec people", while RH says:

> Generally, I find that my being sapphic and in a relationship with a woman makes people (including queer people, friends, family) assume I'm an allosexual gay woman and that must be

> it. If it comes up, I might correct them, but for most people my queerness automatically erases my a-spec-ness, even after knowing I'm a-spec.

When asked if they considered themselves to be part of the LGBTQ+ community, the only people I spoke to who said "no" did so because they had personally not felt welcome in those spaces: RK, for example, answered, "Not really. We don't get a letter," and DE, "I know intellectually that I am (and will tell other people that asexual people are part of the LGBTIA+ community) but sometimes I feel like I personally am not part of it. (I know I am, though, so this is my own thing.)" LV said:

> I wanted to for a long time but I never felt welcome. With the constant a-spec exclusionism and general sentiment that we're not queer enough, I stopped wanting to be included. I also got a ton of harassment from LGBT+ members who were exclusionists.

RR said:

> I'm aware that some LGBT+ people don't believe that a-spec people (that aren't in some other way connected) deserve to be a part of the community because they haven't faced enough oppression, which is an ironic statement. However, I know that other parts of the community are lovely and absolutely support ace identities.

NT, who is both ace and a transgender woman, said outright that "Allo Queers are often worse than Cis-Het folks – certainly so when it comes to inclusion in Queer spaces. Don't even get me started on being Trans Ace with the Cis Allo Queer community..."

For my interviewees, despite their easy accessibility, and the fact that for many of us who live outside urban centres they were our first queer communities, *online* queer spaces seemed especially toxic. A number of people I spoke to explicitly differentiated between positive experiences at in-person, inclusive queer events and spaces, versus outright harassment, erasure and otherwise aphobic commentary they'd encountered in online spaces.

For GH, the online queer community *was* the community. When asked if she considered herself a part of it, she said, "Not really. Twitter is already a particularly nasty place, and I don't really need to deal with aphobic comments disregarding and disparaging our existence." EL echoed this, saying, "one of the side effects of all of the discourse online (2015ish on Tumblr, happening a lot now on Twitter) is that I don't inherently trust that LGBTQ communities will be welcoming."

Rather than disavowing and then dismissing this pattern of aphobia within allo LGBTQ+ spaces, I wanted to look more closely at where it comes from. I wanted to understand what would cause someone in my community, who I might otherwise consider a comrade in arms, to treat someone like myself with outright hostility.

A great deal of this comes from the history of the gay rights movement, and from the way that sex and sexuality have been policed, weaponised specifically against allosexual LGBT+ people throughout Western history. Queers have been fined, imprisoned or even killed because of who we have sex with, since even before "homosexual" or "queer" were constructed as identities. The ability to fuck in peace and safety has been a rallying point – often a life-or-death struggle – for the queer community for as long as that community has existed,[8] and despite the victories of decriminalisation and marriage equality in many Western countries, there are still many places in the world where homosexuality is punishable by fines, imprisonment or even death.

And just as the assertion of women's sexual agency, and the status of a woman as sexual in her own right regardless of the presence of a man, has been a cause around which feminists have organised for decades, demands from the queer community to be able to love who we love, and fuck freely in safety and dignity, have created within most LGBTQ+ spaces an atmosphere of radical, often compulsory, sex positivity.

This attitude, in turn, has led to a perception within these spaces that equates asexual and aromantic ways of being, as far as they involve an *absence* of visible queer sex or queer coupling, with the kind of anti-sex moral conservatism associated with the persecution of allo queers.[9]

What this means for a-spec people is that an *appearance* of normativity is mistaken for actual normativity. In many queer spaces – especially the clubs and bars around which so much of queer culture has by necessity coalesced – there's an implicit, or even explicit, assumption that if you are not actively loving (or fucking) queerly, you do not belong.

HD recalls reading:

> a post a (gay) man wrote about how it was unfair for asexual people to try and date allosexual (I believe he actually said "normal") gay people because gay people already have enough trouble trying to find partners and it wasn't fair for someone who didn't want to have sex to take up their time without disclosing their sexuality.

This sense of outsiderhood within the LGBTQ+ community doesn't always take the form of the outright aphobia that HD experienced. Megan Milks, one of the editors of *Asexualities: Feminist and Queer Perspectives*, says in the introduction:

> Within queer communities as within straight ones, I found myself alienated by the emphasis placed on sex and the pursuit of sex, especially as a single person whose nonsexual intimacies continually got trumped and displaced by my friends' sexual ones.[10]

K.J. Cerankowski, the other editor of *Asexualities*, discusses their experience of being genderqueer, AFAB and romantically interested in women, but nonetheless feeling out of place because of their asexuality: "I felt like more of a queer ally than a queer member of the group, despite feeling so queer myself."[11]

JH, one of my interviewees, recalls:

> I grew up in a gay-friendly household, read a lot of gay books, found myself gravitating toward gay culture, and still didn't recognise for a long time that I had a place in that culture. I felt like an interloper for so long because I was so disconnected from my own interest/desire/feelings/whatever.

EH echoes this sense of feeling like an interloper within queer spaces, saying that,

> for about two years I was convinced that I was straight, and that I was just being attention seeking (even though I hadn't told anyone) and looking to be part of something I wasn't a part of. It felt, to me, disrespectful on actual LGBTQ+ people to be thinking I was part of the community when I was actually straight. I think the difficulty for me was that, because asexuality is a lack of attraction, it was really weird cos like, I wasn't sexually attracted to women, so I must be straight, right? (Obviously at the time, I didn't quite realise that being straight meant actually being attracted to men, but heteronormativity had me unconsciously setting straight as the default.)

The environment of radical, compulsory (queer) sex positivity, where sex and relationships are often both a key topic of conversation and a site of group bonding, leaves many a-spec people feeling excluded or alienated. The a-spec people I spoke to were themselves keenly aware of the same tension I became aware of after that Pride march, between the huge importance of the queer community as a haven for *all* marginalised experiences of sexuality, attraction and desire, and the history of the criminalisation of queer *sex* specifically. A number of people articulated this tension when discussing their own complex or ambivalent relationships to the queer community.

AB, the person who first told me about the presence of asexual people in the gay rights movement, made note of the unique intersectional nature of the problem:

> It can be challenging as any queer identity has their own unique viewpoints, struggles and issues. The LGBTQ community thus has to manage various matters at once. This can and has resulted in conflicts among queer people but that also hasn't stopped them from working together during all these years. The diversity and the intercommunity relationship are what make the queer community powerful.
>
> Those differences can be frustrating as both parties will never fully understand each other. A lot of misinformed allos want to question our right to be a part of the community or completely deny our identity or struggles; this can result in a lot of tension and harmful stigma and is something that needs to be acknowledged and worked on.

JH agreed, saying:

> There is definitely still the presumption of allosexuality in the

> LGBT community, for sure. And from a certain perspective I have a lot of understanding for why that's been the case. When for such a swath of history sex was criminalized, I can understand holding sex up as a tool and symbol of freedom. But the fact remains that that leaves a lot of people feeling alienated.

JK, when describing xyr experiences as both agender trans and a-spec, said:

> It's been mixed. I've seen more acceptance for ace people as part of the LGBT community but there are questions about cishet aces and I tend to have them as well because I know cisheterosexual does not equal cisheteromantic...but there are still differences that cishet aces have from LGBT aces that make me somewhat careful about the way they can engage with the LGBT community. However, because I do know that there is a previous history of asexuals in general counting (i.e. among LGB and T), I'm okay with asexuals participating...

There are also some aspects of mainstream LGBTQ+ activism that may inadvertently lead to some members of the community being erased. The "born-this-way" narrative, which asserts queer desire and identity as both stable and permanent, has been instrumental in the fight against harmful stereotypes of queerness as a "fad" or phase, and the dangerous perception that it can be cured.[12] But there are plenty of people within the community whose experiences of sexuality, gender, desire or attraction are *not* stable. EF, for example, describes the journey they went on before coming to identify as aroace:

> I identified as a lesbian when I realised that aroace fit me so much more. For me, it was very difficult. I felt like a complete

> fraud to go from identifying as gay to identifying as ace, as though I'd been lying to everyone, that I'd gone through a "phase".

"Born-this-way" language risks alienating or even erasing people whose sexualities or genders are fluid or developing – a category that includes many a-spec people, but also a vast array of allo queers as well. In many ways, just like in the straight world, the presence of a-spec people can be contentious because it challenges conventional party lines.

This is one of the dangers of assimilationist activism: several times while I was working on this book I would become aware of the way a community's fight for mainstream acceptance might end up throwing people whose stories don't fit the narrative under the bus.

A-spec people have always been here. Our lived experiences cannot be fully disentangled from allo queer folks', and our political goals are by no means mutually exclusive. The hetero-patriarchal system demanding we all must and may only have hetero-, married, vanilla sex also says men are men and women are women, and never the twain shall meet. It is the system that says you must couple up, it must be with the right people, and it must be within a socially and legally validated contract.

Nothing about the inclusion of a-spec people in LGBTQ+ spaces in any way erases what allo queers have faced, and our inclusion can only strengthen the community. But in order for the queer community, which includes us whether anyone wants it to or not, to be called truly inclusive, some of the politically convenient fictions we've created will have to change. Any future vision that advocates for everyone to be able to love who they love, and have sex in safety and freedom, but that *doesn't* allow the possibility of a happy, healthy, fulfilled asexual, aromantic, demi or grey-a existence is inherently flawed. Freedom *from* is an essential part of freedom *to*: without the first, the second cannot truly exist.

Discussion questions

1. If you have experience moving in LGBT+ spaces, have you seen a-spec identities represented within those spaces? If so, in which contexts? Were a-spec people represented more strongly online or in person? At Pride events? In university-based LGBT+ spaces? Think about where you've seen (or not seen) a-spec people represented in queer communities, and why this might be.
2. If you are on the ace spectrum, do you or have you in the past considered yourself to be part of the LGBT+ community? Is this *because* you are a-spec, or because you are part of another queer subgroup such as the trans or bi/pan communities? Have your experiences, and your feelings about your own place in the LGBT+ community, changed over time?
3. If you are a-spec, how comfortable do you feel moving within LGBT+ spaces?
4. If you are LGBT+ and allosexual/alloromantic, how do you feel about the idea of a-spec people taking up space in the LGBT+ community? Where do you think your attitudes and feelings come from?

Intersectionality

One of the most important lessons I learned while putting this book together was that ace-spectrum identity is highly intersectional – in other words, a person's individual experience of being ace, aro, demi or grey-a can be very different depending on all the other facets that make us who we are.

Because I am white, and because I was very online when I first started getting to grips with my (a)sexuality, it was relatively easy for me to access the language of the community, and to start seeing myself as part of it. Most of the a-spec people I had seen so far, in profile pictures and photos, looked like me, more or less. But for Yasmin Benoit – the aroace activist and model I mentioned in the chapter on visibility, who had never met another Black a-spec person until an in-person LGBT Pride event – things weren't so simple. The invisibility of a-specs of colour was part of what prompted Benoit to start the #thisiswhatasexuallookslike movement: for a young aroace person who'd only ever seen the white face of the community, for someone living outside Anglophone American online culture, for a Native American a-spec whose only access to LGBT Pride events or community spaces might be via a smartphone, encountering that hashtag might be as life-changing as first discovering the community at all, a necessary part of becoming visible to themself and others.

Aside from questions of visibility, your experiences of moving through the world as a-spec can be drastically different depending on the expectations and assumptions people make about you, especially concerning sex and sexuality, family and reproduction.

Because of the way sex especially has been policed and politicised, particularly over the last few hundred years, stereotypes have emerged – or been created – that paint certain demographics as more or less "inherently sexual", in spite of the obvious fact that sexuality is individual. No person is more or less likely to *be* ace or a-spec based on where they come from or who their ancestors were, in the same way no one is more or less likely to be gay – though personal circumstances can dictate whether they are able to be visible, and how the people around them react to their identity. Nonetheless, people of colour, and disabled aces, for example, routinely find that the assumptions others make about them – be that to desexualise or hypersexualise them – erase their asexuality, allowing no space for it to exist as an individual identity.

Asexuality and aromanticism too may pose different challenges, even dangers, depending on personal context. As a visibly queer, trans person already active in LGBTQ+ spaces, coming out as ace and arospec has posed challenges, but it hasn't completely shattered the ground the rest of my identity is based on. Cisgender men, however, are expected (in the West at least) to perform a specific kind of aggressive sexuality as part of their *gender* performance. Much more than for women and queers, asexuality may challenge the very foundations of a cis man's gender identity and may put him at risk of exclusion or even violence from his peers.

In the sections that follow, I'll explore some of the unique challenges faced by the a-spec people I spoke to and heard from

– the ways their experiences of being a-spec were complicated by their gender, cultural background and experience of racialisation and of pathologisation outside asexuality.

Before I go on, I want to state clearly: I come from an American WASP background, and I'm not a race scholar. There are many a-spec BIPOC writers and academics who have studied these topics in depth, whom I will reference throughout this chapter, and I provide suggestions for further reading at the end of the book. I'm also not disabled, though I am neurodivergent.

Throughout this chapter generally, whenever the discussion didn't relate to my own lived experience, I've tried to foreground the voices and experiences of the people I spoke to. In addition, I want to stress that while I'm exploring ways in which my interviewees' and other real people's experiences were shaped by their cultural or racial backgrounds, every single person's experience is different, and just because two people share intersections of identity that doesn't mean their experiences will be the same.

Cultural background and racialisation

Note: This section contains discussion of genocide and the transatlantic slave trade, as well as passing mentions of sexual abuse and forced sterilisation.

CW, one of my oldest friends, has known she is queer for a long time, but only recently came out as ace. We spoke about the complications of "dating while ace", and she mentioned the way other people's perceptions of her as a Black woman, even a queer Black woman, rendered her asexuality invisible:

> It's really really interesting, considering Black women, Black

> femmes, are painted with this "hypersexualisation" paintbrush. And here I am like, "nah", and people have a really hard time conceptualising that. They're like "that doesn't make any sense... you're not doing the prescribed thing for you." And it's like, yeah I am. It's my personal prescribed thing. And it's ever-evolving. So you can't tell me what I should and shouldn't be doing, based on my skin tone. Screw you.
>
> You know, the first thing on my dating profile is usually like "Hi, I am asexual," and I've had lots of people being, "no you're not" or "oh that's fake" or "oh, I can change that in a heartbeat." Delete delete block, bye! Fuck off. So, it's...really rather interesting, and a little fascinating just to see people being people. And a little frustrating. A lot frustrating, let's be real.

CW met the erasure of her identity with defiance and humour, but her frustration and disillusionment came through as well. Her experiences were echoed by JK, who is grey-aro and ace, and uses the words agender, trans or gender fugitive to describe xyr relationship with gender. JK spoke about the ways Black sexuality has been constructed in popular consciousness (which includes a-spec spaces), and the ways the language of asexuality has been shaped specifically around a *white* ace identity:

> I do identify as part of the African diaspora and that certainly interacts with my a-spec identity because I come from a group of people often oversexualized or desexualized as a result of the history of being enslaved and so that kind of continues to impact how people see people from my diaspora to this day...
>
> I often find myself understanding my a-spec identity differently because of my cultural identity and have less patience for some terms and understandings of sexuality that come from white aces as a result.

When discussing xyr experiences specifically within the a-spec community, JK said xyr ability to move comfortably was dependent on the visible presence of other Black a-spec people:

> I have fond memories of hanging out with the Transyadas (a group of nonbinary AVEN users) on the AVEN forum since they helped me make sense about my asexuality and my lack of gender around the same time. And I did make some neat internet acquaintances through that.
>
> But the overall experience has left me kind of...alienated from most ace communities. If it's not specifically for Black aces...I don't really care to be there. Or at the bare minimum – ace people of colour, but even then...I would demand specific places for Black aces there too. So that's where I'm coming from.

When asked if xe had any future hopes for the a-spec community, or changes xe would like to see, JK said:

> More involvement in connecting Black aces together. And connecting aces of colour. Otherwise, the white people need to get their racist ass behaviour together. But I'm not expecting that to happen any time soon.

Xyr hopes for the community centred around connection and coalition between Black aces and aces of colour, and xyr words suggest a perception that the racism within the community is too entrenched to truly be rooted out.

This perception of whiteness – and the presence of racism – within the community is not a coincidence. People growing up right now are more than ever able to access both the language and spaces of the a-spec community. But this access is not distributed evenly.

From its beginning, the language of asexuality and aromanticism, the language I use and celebrate in this book, have been mostly articulated within spaces that are white and Anglophone. This is because the spaces where our terminology started to come together for the first time in their present form were spaces that, considering the distribution of internet access in the 1990s and early 2000s, were already predominantly white and economically privileged.[1]

The people who were in a position to assert their asexuality – aromanticism and other spectrum identities were not yet articulated as such – and take up visible space in the community "looked" (and still look) a certain way. Out of the slew of daytime talk show interviews with ace people that took place in the early 2000s, the vast majority were white,[2] and today, most mainstream pop culture representation of "asexual" people – from BBC's *Sherlock* to Sheldon from *Big Bang Theory* to "that one episode" of *House* – is white as well.

So despite the egalitarian atmosphere within our spaces, our language and community were only accessible to a limited subset of people from the outset – which means that today, the visible face of the a-spec community is a white, technologically literate one. There is still a strong perception, both inside the community and out, that asexuality is a "white thing".[3]

This creates a discomfort for a-spec people of colour like CW and JK when trying to take up space in that community, and it means that the people who *do* feel comfortable – those who've been present from the start – continue to take up space and tell their stories disproportionately to others. It also means that the complexities of the ways race and culture shape the a-spec experience have, for the most part, gone un-talked about.

This has started to change, thanks in large part to the concerted efforts of Black and Indigenous a-specs and a-spec people of colour – researchers, writers, creatives and activists – who have risked the dangers associated with visibility to make their voices heard. Media representation, too, is starting to change, with more authentic representative works being created, crucially by a-specs themselves, that feature the full range of diversity of the community.

In 2021, the main period of time in which I wrote this book, AceCon had dedicated panel tracks broadcast on YouTube, where (possibly thanks to the pandemic) a-spec panellists from all over the world were able to take part and share their experiences.

It was through reading and listening to the words of BIPOC a-spec people, and those from outside the Anglophone West, that I was able to gain a deeper understanding of the ways a person's background can influence everything from what is expected of them romantically and sexually by others in their community, to how and when they are able to explore and unpack their own sexuality and orientation, to how they are permitted to engage with sexuality and desire within a globalised system of white heteropatriarchy.

The people I spoke to in depth for this project came from an astonishing array of cultural backgrounds. Many of them were not white, and while all of them needed English to be able to communicate with me, not all would consider themselves primarily Anglophones.

The communities we grow up and spend most of our time in have a huge influence on the language and spaces we are given access to, and when and in what way we are first able to engage with sexual and romantic desire. For many people, these factors determine not only when and if they are able to find their way to the a-spec community but also how their a-spec identity is received by the people around them, and at what point that identity becomes (if it ever does) not just a description of experience but a *place of marginalisation*.

A number of the people I spoke to in depth for this project said they had grown up Christian, especially Catholic, and so had encountered the idea of celibacy early in life. In *Ace*, Angela Chen discusses Christian purity culture, framing Christian concepts of celibacy not as a progressive acceptance or tacit approval of non-sexual ways of being, but rather as a symptom of a specifically religious brand of compulsory sexuality.[4] Celibacy occupies part of a larger system of penance and sacrifice,[5] considered fundamentally inimical to "natural" human existence, and therefore exceptional. Sexual abstinence is a transcendent quality – pious – precisely because, in a Christian worldview, sex is assumed to be a universally human drive.

It's easy to see, then, why so many of our experiences within Christianity are deeply ambivalent. JH, who, while critical of the religious institution still considers herself to be Catholic, says:

> Oh ho ho ho. So obviously Catholics have a very specific relationship to sexuality and the body. At times I've been comforted by it – see? I'm not doing this wrong! – even while knowing objectively that by any of their very incorrect measures I am doing it wrong. I'm not saving myself for marriage. I won't procreate. I'm not going to become a nun and devote myself to God. So while it might be comforting sometimes to find meaning in the lives of the virgin martyrs, that comfort comes from a deeply problematic place. And I hate that.

LM, who is Christian as well as aroace, says:

> I know my asexuality doesn't come from my Christianity – even in Christian circles, asexuality as an orientiation isn't very well

> known – but never being interested in sex is not really seen as a good thing. Churches speak of marriage as God's plan for everyone, and that sex is God's gift to married couples. By not being interested in sex, there's an implication that I'm rejecting God's gift, his plan for my life.

CD, too, had a lot to say about her experience of growing up in a conservative Catholic community, and a deep understanding of the complex relationship between celibacy and (a)sexuality. When asked whether the interaction between her religious background and her ace and demiromantic identities was positive or negative, CD said:

> ...mixed; when I was young, after my abuse made me feel strongly that I was not suited for marriage (lots of bad baggage from the religious perspective), I sought to join a convent, since it seemed like the option that was left available to me. That said, it also felt like a good option at the time – a positive effect of Catholicism's high regard for virginity is the continued existence of single-sex communities, and I feel like I would have been a good fit in some ways.

She added:

> Catholicism generally places a very high value on chastity and virginity; living a "consecrated single life" (whether or not that means actually becoming a member of a religious order) is considered the most sacred of vocations. It is what Christ was considered to have been, and is a condition still imposed upon priests. That said, it is difficult to map the Catholic concept of a vocation onto a sexual identity.

LG, for their part, had a rather glib take on Christian ideas around chastity, summing up the inherent contradiction at the heart of Christian purity culture, and the pointlessness of trying to equate chastity and asexuality: "I'm not religious but sometimes I like to laugh at the idea that me being a forever virgin would make me extra pure in Christian eyes. Too bad I masturbate though RIP guess I'm a slut after all."

Cultural taboos around sex, too, mean asexuality might go unremarked; an AFAB grey-aroace person like LG, who grew up in Greece where there are taboos around sexuality for young women, might not experience outright discrimination – instead, their asexuality was rendered completely invisible. LG recalled that, growing up, it was actually their aromanticism rather than their asexuality that marked them out: "I experienced some strife over my friends being infatuated and getting crushes and me not being the same. Well thankfully due to sex being taboo for girls I didn't experience the same thing with being asexual."

Nonetheless, they found themself at a tense intersection of conflicting values. When asked how their gender interacts with their experience of being aro and ace, LG, who uses nonbinary and demi-woman to describe their gender, described being simultaneously forbidden to engage with sex but nonetheless perceived in a sexual way by others:

> Greece, the place I grew up in, is some decades behind when it comes to certain social issues, feminism included. There's a lot of sexism and objectification of women. As an ace teen girl that sort of thing made me so uncomfortable. It was just a constant reminder that in male eyes this is how they see and want to see my body. I have always been uncomfortable with being sexualised (as most women, I assume) but as an ace person it just adds another layer of discomfort. And yet another that it

> was assumed that due to being a shy and quiet person it would translate into me needing a man to take the reins and that I would most likely be sexually submissive as well. This was not so much something that was directly said to me (except for one shitty ex-friend) but it's the impression I got from society. It makes me really uncomfortable that someone would perceive me as sexual and even more so if they were to make invasive assumptions on how I would be in bed based on innocuous behaviours of mine.

LG's discomfort reminds me of conversations I'd had with sex-repulsed asexuals, whose repulsion was associated with being perceived as a sexual being, active or passive, by others. For an a-spec person living in communities where this type of non-consensual sexualisation is highly normalised, this might be a constant source of shame, stress or even trauma. And these communities need not be ones that are seen, as LG puts it, as "behind the times" on social issues; LG also recounted similar experiences within LGBTQ+ spaces, which are widely regarded as highly progressive:

> I get the same feeling of discomfort when I see other LGBT+ people say ridiculous things like "If you keysmash, you're a bottom". Like are we really creating stereotypes based on behaviour the same way cistraight people create gender stereotypes?

Cultural and religious expectations around marriage, child-rearing and family-building were also a source of pressure for many people I spoke to, especially those on the aromantic spectrum. SS, who comes from a Romani background, told me:

> Romani culture puts emphasis on the importance of family and having children. Being asexual, the pressure to have children can

> often feel invasive and invalidating. I do like the idea of having children and being a parent, but my primary concern is that my disability would prevent me from being the kind of parent I want to be regardless of my culture's norms.

SS's words demonstrate the complex intersection between (a)sexuality, gender, (dis)ability and ethnicity. Her words echo Ria, one of the speakers on an AceCon panel of East and Southeast Asian asexuals.[6] Ria, who is from the Philippines, spoke about her family's dismissal of her asexuality and valuing of friendships, and of pressure to continue the family tree: "If you don't have a family at the end of your life, then there's really no point, in their eyes."

In a post titled "Being Aroflux & Black" on the Aurea[7] website, activist Kimberly Butler wrote:

> It always felt like black culture couldn't align much with Aromanticism, especially cause growing up I was taught that marriage was the end goal and that's what I should want but I don't think marriage was in my plans. I would dream of having dogs and living alone in a big house instead of having a romantic partner.

For an a-spec person like myself, who comes from a culture with less of an emphasis on family-building and having kids, asexuality or an unwillingness to have children might not lead to marginalisation in the same way as Ria, SS and Butler experienced.

BH, a devout Mennonite (MCUSA), experienced similar pressure within her religious community:

> It [religion] definitely complicates things. Being a Mennonite

> woman is changing in the twenty-first century, but a huge majority of women in my church are still less educated than men, marry young and have children. People aren't bothered by my singleness, but they nearly always assume I have the goal of finding a man and bearing children. I have to turn down a lot of well-intentioned people who sign me up to help with the children because they presume I'd like to practise caring for them before I have my own. There are (a few) gay and lesbian Mennonites, but even the same-gendered couples I know in the church have all gotten married and adopted children.

When asked about the interaction between her religion and her asexuality, she said:

> Mixed. Because I'm still in my twenties, many people just assume I'm failing at finding a man to marry. Unlike the Catholic church, Mennonite clergy are nearly always married, so there aren't single role models, and being single for a long time is looked down on.

DE, who is aroace and not Christian but Orthodox Jewish, echoed this sentiment, and further how she had employed her understanding of religious custom to carve space for herself as a single woman:

> It is a cultural (religious) norm that people want to get married and have children. A large portion of Orthodox women start dating when they are 20. I find it very helpful to point out that women have no obligation by Torah law to be married or have children (the obligation for this commandment is on men instead), though people don't really understand why I wouldn't want to get married and have children anyway.

The pressure placed on us as individuals, to have kids and raise families, doesn't always come from a neutral place, either. A community's history can inform the way the people in it conceptualise sex, romance and obligations around family and parenthood, especially in light of generational trauma.

In 2021, researchers published a paper in *Child Trends* titled "Family, Economic, and Geographic Characteristics of Black Families with Children 2021".[8] The authors draw a direct link between institutional racism in the United States and the experiences and values of Black Americans surrounding family and coupledom: "Culturally, Black Americans have long highly valued romantic partnerships, marriage, and children. However, institutional and structural barriers often prevent them from being able to realize these values." In other words, America's history of white supremacy plays a heavy role in shaping Black Americans' experiences of romance, sexuality, desire and family-building. It's not much of a leap to surmise that this history and context might provide an additional barrier to Black a-spec people, such as Butler, in discovering and expressing their identities, especially if that expression involves rejecting the trappings of marriage and nuclear family.

In the AceCon panel about the experiences of Indigenous a-spec people in North America,[9] one of the audience questions was: "Have there been differences in the way the wider dominant (read: white) culture has dealt with your asexuality versus your specific Indigenous cultures?"

Johnnie Jae's answer to this question consciously linked her community's history, of violent colonisation at the hands of white settlers and the US government, to her experience as an asexual person in that community today:

> There's so many expectations that are put on female-presenting

> people in terms of what our role in our community is... We're [Indigenous North Americans] less than 2 per cent of the US population and with this pandemic it's possible that we are going to go back to under 1 per cent because of how hard our communities have been hit. And so there is a lot of pressure now to, you know, create those "pandemic babies"... It's not a very good conversation to have, when you're asexual or you don't identify as female or male, or you're within the LGBTQIA community, because there are a lot of people who do feel that we are contributing to our own genocide. And that's a heavy, heavy accusation to deal with. Because you understand where they're coming from and why they think this, but at the same time, it is still so violent and inappropriate to put that burden on people who...we can't help who we are, and we shouldn't have to force ourselves into these other roles or be expected to just for the sake of survival.

The ramifications of one community being denied sexual and reproductive agency at the hands of another have far-reaching consequences. In the context of a community still dealing with the repercussions of genocide, ethnic cleansing, forced sterilisation or any other form of violence directly leading to a reduced population – many of which are still happening today to communities around the world – any a-spec person unable or unwilling to "do their part" in what others around them might see as "rebuilding the community" might experience a marginalisation of their a-spec identity in a very specific way – a way not experienced by their peers from dominant racial and ethnic groups.

For an a-spec person in these communities, coming out cannot be as simple as just "opting out" of the institutions of marriage, sex and nuclear family. This complexity may simultaneously limit that person's ability to apply a-spec language to themself, and render them doubly invisible once they do join the community, especially if family and reproductive pressure are forces they cannot simply shrug off.

Expectations around sexuality and family, and pressure to perform sexuality and desire in a certain way, do not always come from within your own community, either. In fact, the conclusion this section has been circling towards is the idea that the most profound force influencing how and whether a person can own their asexuality or aromanticism may not be cultural background, but race, or more specifically racialisation.[10]

The experiences of BIPOC a-spec people show us the ramifications of the way human sexuality has been weaponised in order to maintain the status quo. For most asexual, aromantic, demi and grey-a people of colour, simply existing as themselves, in light of this history, is a revolutionary act.

Racial justice activist Paul Kivel writes, "Whiteness is a constantly shifting boundary separating those who are entitled to have certain privileges from those whose exploitation and vulnerability to violence is justified by their not being white."[11]

One of those sets of privileges has long been access to sexual and reproductive agency. In her essay "On the Racialisation of Asexuality",[12] Ianna Hawkins Owen unpacks a particularly pertinent and far-reaching example: American chattel slavery.

Through looking at the twin stereotypes of the sexually aggressive, dangerous "Jezebel" and the desexualised-and-therefore-safe "Mammy", Owen explores the way "asexuality", not as an identity but as a quality of sexual restraint, has been positioned as a characteristic of whiteness, associated with concepts of "purity" and "refinement" – in contrast to Black people, who were characterised as "hypersexual" as justification for denying them autonomy and self-rule. This denial, like the rest of the transatlantic slave trade, was economically motivated: controlling the sexual agency of enslaved people, who represented a self-reproducing source of free labour, was a question of finances. With this in mind, Owen traces "the crafting of a sexualized racial threat", in the form of, for example, caricatures of Sarah Baartman, a Khoikhoi woman trafficked to Europe and displayed in highly exploitative and sexualised "exhibits" – and culminating in the creation of "Jezebel" and "Mammy".

Owen concludes with a look at the current-day ramifications of this history. She explores how modern representations of asexuality, commonly seen as a "white thing", influence how white asexuals are treated and perceived, and the relative invisibility of Black asexual people.

Today, the stereotypes of Mammy and Jezebel live on in our cultural consciousness and in pop culture, and they circumscribe the ways that Black women like my friend CW are able to engage with asexuality.

Assumed from even a young age to be sexually mature and assertive,[13] a Black woman may find herself disbelieved in her asexuality, as CW was. If she is middle-aged that ace identity might be dismissed as inconsequential, in light of stereotypes like Mammy, that paint older Black women as non-sexual in the first place. An aromantic Black woman might find her identity weaponised against her, in the form of accusations of "promiscuity". A demisexual Black woman trying to date may find that, more so than a white demi woman, others are likely to disrespect her boundaries around sex.

In the same way that hypersexuality has been used as a tool to limit Black women's sexual and reproductive agency, other demographics have found their sexualities, their ability to experience desire or to be perceived as *desirable*, denied wholesale.

In her essay "(Re)sexualising the Desexualised Asian Male

in the Works of Ken Chu and Michael Joo",[14] Joan Kee states, "The Asian or Asian American male is perhaps best known for his absence in the colonizer's sexual hierarchy." In other words, under the white gaze, Asian men regularly find the existence of their sexuality dismissed, and themselves denied the possibility of possessing romantic or sexual desire, painted as undesirable and therefore undesiring.

And as Kee's quote suggests, just as with Black women, the stereotypical idea of Asian male (non)sexuality links back to colonialism – specifically to white American anxieties around East Asian immigration near the end of the nineteenth century. These fears around an increasingly visible diaspora population led to Asian sexuality, like Black sexuality in the South, coming to be seen as a threat. This anxiety, culminating in the 1882 Chinese Exclusion Act,[15] resulted in consistent media portrayals of Asian men as villainous, threatening, unmanly foreigners – portrayals that have loud echoes in pop culture to this day.[16]

It is this dynamic that writer and performance artist Alok Vaid-Menon writes about in their essay "What's R(ace) Got to Do With It?: White Privilege & (A)sexuality":[17] "Part of white supremacy as I understand it is the privilege of being a subject of desire: one who can feel in control of one's desires and one who has more agency to act on said desires."

Vaid-Menon laments the way this stereotype has denied them the ability to freely identify as asexual, because a visibly non-sexual existence as an Asian person[18] reinforces those stereotypes. As Angela Chen puts it in *Ace*,[19] marginalised people "can find it very difficult to claim asexuality because it looks so much like the product of sexism, racism, ableism and other forms of violence", or in the words of Vaid-Menon: "my asexuality is a site of racial trauma".

The a-spec people I spoke to were aware of this legacy of

desexualisation, and it did often lend an ambivalence to their discussions of a-spec identity. When I asked her thoughts on a-spec representation in popular culture, GH, who is Filipino American, said:

> I'd like to see more aces of color. As of now, we have Alice from *Let's Talk About Love*, who is Black, Emma from *Not Your Backup* is Latinx, and Ellie in *Elatsoe* is Indigenous. I'd like to see an Asian ace in fiction, which I know some would object since Asians, particularly Asian men, are negatively depicted as desexualized. I am currently writing a YA with a Filipino ace main character.

Racialisation is one of the ways that society tells people things about themselves that aren't true. Assumptions around sexuality were baked into the racial hierarchy from the start, right alongside ideas around characteristics like skin colour or hair texture. The sexual dimension *cannot* be separated from the way race has been constructed, because, from the beginning, sexuality and reproduction have gone hand in hand with racist ideas about self-government and "fitness to rule".

To an extent, those of us who were able to assert their asexuality in the early days of the community were able to do so because we were free of the racialised norms and expectations placed on people of colour. Within a larger culture of amatonormativity and compulsory sexuality, no one – especially those of us from marginalised groups – can come to know and love their a-spec self without access to the self-knowledge that comes from community, and freedom from sexual stereotypes. In its current form, without serious work, the a-spec community cannot be a place where everyone can access that self-knowledge.

The more the borders of the a-spec community open up, the more people we allow to take up space here, the more important it will be for us to listen to the least visible members of our community and challenge power dynamics that have until now gone mostly unchallenged. As long as white a-spec people uncritically assert their right to not bear children without acknowledging the privilege allowing them to do so, or claim the language of asexuality without knowing where it comes from, our community cannot truly be said to be a safe and inclusive one.

Discussion questions

1. How do you think your cultural background has shaped your experiences of sexuality and desire?
2. How do you think your race, whether you are white or a person of colour, affects the way other people perceive you? Do people make assumptions about your sexuality or romantic orientation?
3. If you are a-spec, how do you think your race has shaped your experience of your a-spec identity?

Gender

I asked the people I spoke to how they thought their gender affected their experience of being a-spec, but it wasn't until I actually started writing this chapter that it occurred to me to try to answer this question myself.

Nine tenths of the problem, for me, is the fact that I'm not actually sure what my gender is. To a binary-gendered person this might sound ridiculous, but it's true: just like with my sexuality and romantic orientation, my gender stubbornly resists my every attempt to put words to it.

I rely on catch-all terms and signals of political solidarity – trans, nonbinary, queer – but I've given up trying to decide if a word like "genderfluid" or "neutrois" is more accurate. Agender might be the way to go, but if I'm honest I'm not even sure that I *don't* have a gender – it's more that I just don't know what that gender, if it exists, *is*. Perhaps I should say "quoigender", if such a word exists, or use JK's evocative "gender fugitive".

"Gender" as a concept isn't much use to me. For all intents and purposes, my gender only exists as far as it unites me and identifies me with others in my community – that's why "trans" is my favourite word to use, even though it is the broadest term. Transgender people are the people I feel at home with, and whom I want to fight alongside. "Trans" feels right to me as well because it implies transgression, subversion, a gender that challenges why we even *have* a concept of gender in the first place.

It also didn't occur to me until now that perhaps I'd have a better idea of my gender if I had a stronger sense of a sexuality or romantic orientation. After all, so much of what is expected of us as "men" and "women" is tied up in (hetero)sexual, romantic and family-related norms.

As a nonbinary person, I'm "outside" binary gender, one of the most powerful systems acting on all of us, shaping the way we live our lives – and as an a-spec person I'm outside another, closely related system: (compulsory/hetero)sexuality. Without these systems, and without the social scripts that go along with them – telling us who is supposed to propose to whom, who is supposed to be aggressive and who demure, who is supposed to do childcare – gender seems to have nothing to anchor itself upon.

I'm not alone in this gender-confusion. Around 42 per cent of the 15,123 people who answered the "gender" question on the

2020 Ace Census survey listed something other than just "man or male" or "woman or female", instead putting any number of terms such as "genderfluid", "nonbinary", "demigirl", "demiguy", "neutrois" or a combination thereof,[20] or even just "no gender", and while I didn't specifically ask them about their trans status – so there was no way for me to know if someone who listed their gender as "male" was trans or cis – of the 160 or so people who responded to my original Google survey, a whopping 70, nearly half, indicated something other than "(cis) woman" or "(cis) man" in the "gender" box. Thirty-nine of these (like the Ace Census survey, around 24%) specifically put nonbinary or a related identity like genderfluid or neutrois.

Compared to an estimated 0.3 per cent of nonbinary people living in the USA in 2021,[21] the difference is glaring. Within both my and the Ace Census researchers' sample of a-spec people, a person was more likely to be nonbinary – or at least to put something other than just "man" or "woman" – than they were to be a man, and among my interviewees, almost as likely to be nonbinary or trans as a cis woman.

Around 25 per cent answered "yes" or "unsure" to the question "Do you identify as transgender?", and there was also a strong showing of binary trans people among the a-specs who shared their experiences with me, though I couldn't see anything to indicate that, for example, trans women are more likely to be ace than trans men or vice versa, or that there was any correlation between being ace or aro and being any particular trans gender, beyond the fact that a-spec identity and gender-nonconformity seem to go hand in hand.

Of course, binary trans people are also subject to sexualised stereotypes and expectations. Cisnormative society is obsessed with trans people's genitals, for one thing: many of us are regularly asked if we've had "the surgery", and most of the articles about trans people written by cis people have an inordinate and morbid focus on gender confirmation surgery. Trans women especially tend to be fetishised and overly sexualised in pop culture and media depictions,[22] so it's easy to see how, like an ace Black woman, an ace trans woman might find herself disbelieved in her asexuality, or her boundaries around sex disrespected.

At the same time, because sexuality is tied in so closely with embodiment, anything that changes the way a person relates to their own body might complicate their experience of (a)sexuality. HelloKuromi, a trans woman on the AVEN forums who had until recently identified as asexual, wrote in a post that starting hormone replacement therapy (HRT) seemed to have increased her desire for partnered sex:

> I'm a pre-op transgender woman. I have always felt completely asexual because of my body dysphoria. It just has felt like I couldn't imagine being with anyone else or how my body would function if I was. But, all of this has started to change since I began hormones six months ago. Suddenly, I feel more "right" in my body, and even though I still have a *thing* between my legs that I don't like, I somehow have a small desire to be sexual occasionally with a partner. I've basically gone from feeling like just asexual to grey-a, instead.

A number of other users responded with anecdotal evidence, saying they'd experienced the same thing. This experience actually complicates a commonly accepted idea about transition, which is that oestrogen and antiandrogens (the hormone regimen generally prescribed to transgender women) reduce libido, and by extension desire for sex. The experiences of ace trans women like HelloKuromi challenge our assumptions about both trans women and asexual people, and she herself was aware of the marginality of her experience. Discussing her newfound sexual desire, she says, "It's quite welcome actually :) It's still isolating though :(Kinda stinks being a minority within a minority."

Communities of sexual and gender minorities are not mutually exclusive; in many cases they overlap considerably. Moving within the a-spec community seems to make it more likely that a person also moves in the LGBTQ+ community and, to an extent, vice versa. As I discussed in the chapter on the relationship between a-spec identity and queerness, lots of us find out that a-spec identities exist in the first place from the LGBTQ+ community – in other words, the queer community is our first exposure to the a-spec community as well.

When I was exploring both my gender and my sexuality for the first time, the same people were talking about these things – not to say that every nonbinary person was ace or that every ace was nonbinary, but that the groups where these words were being thrown around were two mostly overlapping circles. Without access to the queer community as a bank of knowledge, many people may never get the chance to explore their a-spec identity.

There was a particular kind of ambivalence with which many of the people I spoke to seemed to talk about our genders. In the "How would you describe your gender?" box, I received a number of responses from the glib "*vague hand gesture*", and "Female, because I'm AFAB, but gender is strange and I don't really care," to the concise, "don't have one at the moment," to the thoughtful, "I don't experience feelings about any gender whatsoever or even the concept of gender." One respondent to the 2020 Ace Census survey simply put an emoji, " :/ ".

During a discussion of gender and gender presentation, one of my ace friends, DL, used a term that nicely sums up the way so many of the people I spoke to seemed to relate to gender: "gender apathetic". In fact, gender apathy seems like a logical extension of the apathy so many of my ace interviewees seemed to feel towards sex and sexual activity – and I'll discuss the relationship between gender and sex apathy, and a potential additional complication, neurodivergence, in the next section.

This suggests that there may be a deeper connection between the gender-nonconforming and a-spec communities than just learning definitions and vocabulary, however. NT, when asked how her a-spec identity interacts with her (trans) gender, says (my emphasis):

> I would not have come to know myself as an ace if not for having worked through the issues with being trans – *being trans allowed me to strip myself of the social constructs* I had built to hide my authentic self. Accepting myself meant accepting all of myself.

Considering how, as I'll explore further on in this chapter, tangled up sexual expression is with (binary, cis)gender, it's not hard to see how exploring and embracing oneself as gender-nonconforming, as NT did, might go hand in hand with embracing a sexuality outside the norm, as well.

If asexual cisgender men, for example, are under pressure to hide their asexuality because it threatens their status as men, then trans and gender-nonconforming a-specs have already experienced that rupture: there may be nothing left to tie them to gender at all.

> I think so much of how we think about being a woman is wrapped up in how we are supposed to exist in relationship to the heteropatriarchy. Very gendered clothing for women is meant to constrict and minimise the amount of space we

> take up (which also interacts for me with being fat), and is viewed through the lens of how we are perceived by men. I have always identified as a cis woman, but I've always been a little uncomfortable being perceived as a woman. I think a lot of that discomfort comes from being aroace. I have a hard time defining what womanhood is outside of its relationship to heterosexuality. I have also spent the last few years experimenting with the way I dress, and finding clothes and outfits that I feel like I look good in but that aren't trying to appeal to others. EL

Despite the visibility of asexual men like David Jay, and the bulk of ace "representation" in popular media being antisocial white guys in their twenties and thirties, there is an abiding stereotype that women make up a disproportionate number of the ace population.[23] A quick Google search will find reams of posts on sites like Reddit and Quora, of people asking why it seems like there are more women than men in the community, and accompanying reams of speculation as to why.

Many of the people I spoke to were aware of this perception: JTS, one of the few masculine-identified people who I was able to speak to in more depth, said, "There aren't so many men that openly say that they are asexual sadly."

Are there really more women in the a-spec community than men? My first instinct, on starting this project, was to dismiss the stereotype that women are somehow "naturally" more likely to be ace as just that: a stereotype, not based in fact. But numbers don't lie, do they? Out of the 15,123 people who filled in the "gender" question in the 2020 Ace Census, 61 per cent wrote something that could be construed as feminine (i.e. "female", "woman", "cis woman", "trans woman", "demiwoman", "lesbian", etc.). Comparatively speaking, only 17 per cent wrote anything conceivably masculine, and the answers were a mix of "man or male", trans masculine and nonbinary masculine genders like demiguy or nonbinary trans man. When asked to describe their gender, out of the 160 people who answered my original Google form, 63 per cent listed a feminine gender. Comparatively speaking, only 11 per cent listed a masculine gender.

So where does this apparent imbalance come from? The numbers don't lie, but they may not tell the whole truth, either. Rather than there simply being more ace and a-spec women than men, what seems to be at play here is actually the collision of several social and historical forces, creating an appearance of gender imbalance, when really the problem has more to do with visibility.

To explore where these skewed figures come from, it's necessary to look at the ways that gender, and gender performance, are wrapped up in sexuality, especially the origins of today's social expectations around women's and men's sexualities.

For women, those expectations can be traced back to the ways that ideas about women's sexuality have changed over the past few hundred years, especially the idea of female pleasure and the status of women as sexual agents in their own right.

Before the European Enlightenment, it was thought that in order for a child to be conceived, both male and female partners needed to orgasm[24] – and since the Church was generally adamant that all sexual activity ought to be for purposes of procreation, this meant that a woman's participation, her consent and enjoyment, were considered a necessary part of any "correct" sexual conduct. The existence of a woman's sexuality was taken as a given, on par with a man's – in fact women were often perceived as possessing sexual impulses they were powerless to control.[25]

Around the 1700s, however, Western attitudes towards female pleasure, and toward women as sexual agents, began to change.

As economic centres of power shifted away from the home, women found themselves increasingly barred from those centres of power.[26] During this time, women went from being economic agents in their own right – as they had been in the "cottage industry" model where the home, not the factory, was the centre of production[27] – to simply bodies: sites for male pleasure and tools for the consolidation of male power in the form of heirs.[28]

For our purposes, the upshot of this change was that women stopped being seen as active sexual agents in their own right; instead their sexuality was seen as needing to be regulated and controlled,[29] and as nonexistent without a man's participation.[30] Victorian middle-class women were not seen as capable of pleasure but were instead thought of as "the angel in the house",[31] whose needs were subsumed to her husband's.

In a worldview that doesn't consider women to be sexual beings in the first place, the idea of asexual women as a social category could not exist – and this may account for why most of the so-called "asexual historical figures" we know of today[32] are men: the absence of a man's sexual desire would be notable, a woman's not so much.

The sexual revolution of the 1960s[33] emerged against this backdrop of sexual disempowerment, and much of current feminist activism is based around challenging its lingering effects, many of which stubbornly persist to this day: under the male gaze, women are still simultaneously sexual*ised* and seen as inherently less sexual than men, their sexual pleasure valued less than their ability to give that pleasure to men.[34] One of the biggest feminist projects of the twentieth and twenty-first centuries has been to reclaim women's pleasure and sexual agency, by asserting that women, too, desire sex and have sexual needs.

The sexual revolution and the subsequent feminist "sex wars"[35] have resulted in an environment where sex, sexuality, desire and pleasure are the most pertinent topics of conversation, and where sex positivity – an attitude that embraces human sexuality, taking it as fact that women are equally (and universally) possessed of sexual drive as men – is the norm in progressive circles.

This meant that most of the a-spec people I spoke to found themselves living in environments in which sex positivity had become compulsory sexuality. In *Ace*, Angela Chen describes her complex feelings as an ace woman, bopping to female-led hip hop tracks that position sexual pleasure and prowess as the ultimate expression of female power. Chen sums the situation up neatly when she says, "Conspicuous consumption of sex has become a way to perform feminist politics."[36]

In this new context, where both men and women are universally considered to possess sexual appetites, any unwillingness or reluctance to wholly embrace sex and sexuality become conspicuous.

Ironically, it now becomes possible to truly propose "asexual" as a separate category of person, against this background of compulsory sexuality. As Ela Przybylo puts it in "Masculine Doubt and Sexual Wonder", compulsory sexuality creates "the cultural conditions that make asexuality at once both difficult to imagine and possible to formulate".[37]

In this cultural context, ace women often find themselves obligated to perform sexually when they don't want to, but also being told by older female relatives, who may have grown up with different sexual politics, that it's "natural" for them not to want sex while their husband does. You need only look at American sitcoms featuring married couples, so many of which cast husbands as "horndogs" and wives as mildly unwilling or bored instruments for male satiation.

Interviewee OP recalled that her mother "used to tell me that people exaggerate when they talk about sex, and she herself hated talking about anything remotely sexual". Rather than absolving them from pressure to have sex, comments like these instead position asexuality – any reticence on the part of an ace person – as a problem, a hurdle to be overcome.

Asexual and aromantic women are caught in the middle of a moment of political and social change. Ace women's asexuality is denied in sex-positive contexts, where any way of being that doesn't loudly declaim the existence of women's sexuality for its own sake may be seen as a step back into a repressive past, or even as contributing to the marginalisation of her fellow women, regardless of the lived experience of the ace woman in question.

At the same time, in a society that in many contexts still accepts the idea that women are inherently less sexual than men, a woman's asexuality may be accepted but not considered noteworthy – as HD was told when she came out to her family. Rather than accept that she was asexual, they gave "speeches about how the media was oversexualized and what was portrayed on TV about attraction and relationships was not realistic".

In turn, the same system that desexualises women also actively rewards them for performing their social function as nurturers, family-builders and emotional labourers – a memory of the "angel in the house" echoing down the years. Women are shamed for prioritising careers, hobbies, friendship or creative pursuits over their "familial duties", and aromantic women regularly report experiencing shame and stigma for not pursuing romance, coupledom, marriage and family.[38] An aro woman who has sex for pleasure but doesn't form romantic bonds is simultaneously a "girlboss" and cold-hearted: caught between two conflicting social norms, neither of which has her best interest at heart.

The other piece of the puzzle of gender imbalance in the

a-spec community fits into place when we turn to look at the relationship between masculine gender and heterosexuality.

Men, at least in the Anglophone West, are rewarded for performing an active, aggressive sexuality, a sexuality that is thought to constitute, in large part, what makes a man a man. Without that aggressive performance of sexuality, the gender performance – a man's membership in the category of "man" – becomes threatened.

The gender imbalance in the a-spec community doesn't necessarily suggest that there are more ace woman than men, but instead that it is more difficult for men to break from the sexual norms associated with their gender in order to claim the label of "asexual". Aromanticism, too, is complicated by the strong link between binary gender and norms within relationships, with men's roles being more closely tied to sex, with less of the burden of emotional labour compared to women. As Reddit user IfYoudLike, an aromantic allosexual man, said in a reply to a post asking about the differences between aromantic men and women, "I still felt sexual attraction and never thought that romantic and sexual attraction where [sic] any different."

In her essay "Masculine Doubt and Sexual Wonder",[39] Ela Przybylo interviews three asexual men living in the southern Ontario region in Canada. In her conversations with them, she looks at the ways that the "male sexual drive discourse"[40] – the idea that sexuality is a universal biological impulse that drives men to seek out sexual satisfaction – and the "sexual imperative", which is roughly equivalent to what I've been calling "compulsory sexuality", combine to make asexuality, as Przybylo puts it, "uninhabitable" for men.

Early on, Przybylo discusses the difficulty of seeking out interviewees who identified specifically as *men* and *asexual*: the space where these two identities intersect is a volatile one, and membership in one category challenges membership in the other. Przybylo suggests that this tension may have meant that some potential participants whose lived experience might have been enlightening – people socialised as male but who might not identify as such – might have self-selected, electing not to participate.

Przybylo's interviewees, all of whom were heteroromantic, describe not only feeling obligated to perform sexually for their female romantic partners but also intense pressure to use that social script, performing an aggressive, exaggerated sexuality, to bond with other men.

Przybylo says that "manliness is...bound up with not only having sex but also with ostentatiously performing an interest in sex".[41] In other words, it wasn't so much whether they actually had sex that was necessary to pass as normatively masculine in the group, but whether they were able to perform *sexuality* in the right way. Interviewee Billy, for example, recalled as a teenager "playing along" – performing the role he was expected to, of the sexually desiring young man – with his friends, as they bonded while looking at pornography.

All three of the men Przybylo spoke to described having their status as men questioned, if and when their performances were deemed inadequate: as Billy puts it, "If you're out with a bunch of guys and one of them says 'ooo, look at the butt on that,' you got to 'ooo' or else."[42]

So the lingering double standard that casts women as passive sexual receptacles, without desires of their own, and men as natural sexual aggressors, creates an environment where it is easier for women than for men to recognise themselves as asexual. The "direct connection between sex, sexual performance and what it means to be a man"[43] makes asexuality a potentially dangerous space for a man to visibly occupy – especially a cisgender, heteroromantic man.

My findings seemed to support this: the percentage of transgender, nonbinary and queer (aside from any a-spec identity) men seemed to be much higher among the people I spoke to than in the general population. Out of the 2177 people who selected "man or male" on the Ace Census survey gender question, only 17 per cent selected heteroromantic as their current romantic orientation, and only one person (an aromantic man) selected heterosexual as their sexuality.

The category of "man" is at once privileged, unstable and exclusive, with strict entry criteria that require constant maintenance and performance. The smallness and exclusivity of the category are tied to the history of patriarchy, the way that sexual difference has been used to maintain the status quo and the traditional role of men as procreators.

Asexual men find that their gender and sexual expression are policed by other men, as if a single slip might disqualify them, getting their "man card" revoked. The social norms that punish men for being emotionally vulnerable[44] or acting in a way perceived as feminine[45] are the same norms that see any would-be man who fails to conform to male compulsory sexuality as not a man at all but something else: a failed man, punished accordingly.[46]

So the "riddle" of gender imbalance in the a-spec community has less to do with any biological differences between men and women, or between testosterone- and oestrogen-influenced bodies, and far more to do with who is able to safely embody the identity of asexual.

This means many asexual men remain invisible, unable to publicly own their asexuality without totally disrupting their lives *as men*: they risk giving up privilege but also potentially safety. When they *do* come out, they tend to be hypervisible and met with incredulity and disbelief: as Joy Behar said in a 2006 interview with AVEN founder David Jay, "I don't get this. A guy. I could see for a woman. But you? You have to do something."

Any given man's identification with asexuality clashes directly with what society requires of him in light of his status as a man. But I also have hope that, as the definitions and norms around what it means to be a man change, developing alongside our understandings of sex and gender, the numbers will start to change.

Discussion questions

1. How has your gender shaped your experiences of sexuality, desire and attraction, and vice versa?
2. Do you find that other people (or you yourself) have expectations of you to do with sexual and romantic performance? What about within relationships? Family-building?
3. How easy or hard do you find it to go against these expectations?
4. Where do you think these expectations come from?
5. How do you think your experiences might be different if you were a different gender?

Disability, mental illness and neurodivergence

Note: this section contains mentions of aphobic discrimination, corrective rape and childhood sexual abuse.

> Due to autism and dyslexia being innate neurological differences, they play a part in how my brain is wired. While dyslexia affects my ability to read and write, autism affects how I observe, think and socialise, making it the most dominant feature I have. It plays a huge part in how I identify. HI

In the introduction to this book, I mentioned the way that, considering how modern biomedical science has given us a worldview where human beings are slotted into different biological "types", asexuality has for much of modern history been misinterpreted as a disease, an untenable state – and asexual people as broken, lacking and in need of a cure.

The difficulty that so many a-spec people have in coming to understand and embrace themselves as they are comes from the way that pathologisation – the transformation of human variation into illness – muddies the water. Like racialisation and racial stereotypes about sexuality and romance, pathologisation is a way that society tells us things about ourselves that aren't true: namely, that there is something wrong with us that needs curing.

The intersection of asexuality, aromanticism, illness and pathology is a complex and often fraught one. This is because despite the fact that asexuality and aromanticism are not indicative of illness, there are people among us who *are* ill, and because asexuality is not the only identity that has been pathologised in this way.

Stereotypes abound: the idea that "asexuals are just depressed", or "your asexuality is because you're traumatised and don't know it", are misconceptions that aces have to counter daily. At the same time, those of us who are both ace *and* mentally ill, ace *and* medicated, or ace *and* traumatised, often find ourselves silenced or shunted aside within community discourses,[47] in favour of the hard-fought party line that our identities have nothing to do with pathology, and claims that "the plumbing still works".[48]

A number of the people I spoke to fit that description, and in many cases, their a-spec identity *could not be entirely separated* from their experience of illness or trauma – which were often intertwined. RH, for example, who is demiromantic, quoiromantic and aceflux, says, "I originally adopted the label aceflux when I found that my mental health condition and medication was affecting my sexual attraction and sex drive." RH didn't mention that her experiences of illness had necessarily been silenced within the a-spec community, but did say that she has "actively avoided telling medical professionals I am a-spec".

HBJ, who has been diagnosed with chronic clinical depression, said:

> Some of the medications I've taken have killed my libido utterly in the past, and I didn't actually like that, because sexual appetite is not the same as sexual attraction. Depression of course makes it hard to be interested in much of anything, including sex, and can really mess with relationships because you're not able to give any energy to your partner or the relationship in general. But I don't feel that I'm asexual because of my depression, nor depressed because of my orientation.

CD, for her part, related the way her experiences of childhood sexual abuse, leading to severe PTSD, interacted with her asexuality (my emphasis):

> For more than a decade, *the illness sort of covered my asexuality*, if that makes sense – I assumed that my lack of feeling had resulted from my experiences. But with time, and improved mental health, I was able to separate the two, to consider the "data points" indicating that I'd been disinterested in sexual matters even before my bad experiences. (I came home weeping after a school lecture

> on conception, etc., that was mandatory attendance when I was eleven – I asked my parents if there were any other ways to have children. Bless them, they thought it was hilarious!)

When asked if she had any experience with mental illness, CD explicitly mentioned her PTSD as a barrier to her acceptance of her own asexuality: "I do; for a long while, I assumed that – due to my PTSD – I was 'frigid', rather than that I was just myself."

A number of people had experiences with mental illness that they specifically connected to their a-spec identity, with a few even going so far as to say that being a-spec made their mental health worse. But once I had read their words more closely, it soon became clear that it's not a-spec identity itself causing mental illness, but marginalisation stress, and internalised shame and aphobia. AB, for example, said:

> When I was forcing myself to perform heteronormativity, and in that sense erasing my own identity by pretending to be straight, I caused myself a lot of anxiety, panic attacks and it worsened my depression. Especially when I was younger, not accepting myself the way I am is what caused me a lot of stress and trauma.

HBJ too described the way that accepting herself as asexual actively improved her mental health:

> I live with chronic clinical depression and dealt with a lot of misplaced guilt and fear growing up, and a sense that there was something wrong with me. Understanding that asexuality is a real and valid orientation has helped me tremendously to understand that there's nothing wrong with not seeing people in a sexual way.

The complexity of the relationship between asexuality and illness or trauma, combined with the fact that the a-spec community spends so much time asserting that illness and trauma are *not* part of our story, runs the risk of alienating those of us who are both – a vulnerable subset of an already vulnerable group, whose experiences I'll discuss in more depth in the section on sex repulsion in the chapter "Sex".

The silencing of those who have been labelled as both "asexual" and "ill" works in two dimensions: the other side of the coin relates to disability and the disabled community. Both a-spec people who are disabled and disabled people who are a-spec routinely find themselves marginalised within their own communities,[49] and the reasons for this bring us back to the way our society draws such a close association between sexuality, health and social functioning.

I've spoken before about the ways that colonised people have throughout history found their sexuality denied because it was inconvenient to those in power, for example in the case of Asian men. Disabled people have experienced a similar trajectory: for as long as that association between sex and health has existed, disabled people have been framed as undesirable – and therefore *undesiring*.

In this way, disabled people as a community have been desexualised, given the label "asexual" – and by extension "aromantic" – without their consent, and their sexual, romantic and reproductive agency has been curtailed as a result. The disabled community has therefore been tirelessly campaigning for access to sex education[50] and sexual services themselves[51] for decades – and part of these campaigns has involved asserting that disabled people experience sexual and romantic attraction "as much as anyone else".

Under these circumstances, it's easy to see why the existence of asexual-identified disabled people – unwilling to participate in the active sexuality and desire the disabled community has fought so hard to assert – might find themselves marginalised; like ace women within feminist circles, the very fact of their identities is often misinterpreted as undermining the community's fight for liberation.

A number of writers from the disabled community have explored this complex history and the ways it has, so far, undermined the possibility of coalition and solidarity between the a-spec and disabled communities.[52] The conflict between these communities has meant that their considerable overlap in lived experience has long ignored, crucially, their shared history of marginalisation via the biomedical establishment.

The picture beginning to emerge is that, while there is no *inherent* connection between disability and asexuality – and asserting this connection without taking into account ace and disabled peoples' lived experiences does real harm – the two communities are united by the way a "scientific" model of sexuality and desire has been used to cast them both as deficient and subhuman, and deny them the basic dignity of sexual freedom.

It's also essential to understand that, while both communities have been assigned negative value by a society that sees them as broken, neither a-spec identity nor what we call disability are inherently bad or wrong. Instead, they are simply different ways of looking at, or existing in, the world. They only become illnesses, pathologies, problems when that world doesn't make space for or accommodate them.

This understanding has been very important to another, adjacent community: that of neurodivergent, especially autistic, people, who have campaigned for years against the classification of autism as a medical diagnosis.[53] A number of my interviewees said they considered themselves to be neurodivergent, especially with ADHD and autism, two neurodiversities that often coincide,[54] so the experiences of neurodivergent a-spec people are important to bring up.

Just like with the disabled community, the label of "asexual" has been used to infantilise and disempower people with autism.[55] Unlike with disability, however, there have actually been studies that suggest a positive correlation between autism specifically and a-spec identity[56] – though *not* necessarily a causation. At most, there seems to be a significant overlap between these communities, or more precisely between asexuality and autism, and I could find no formal studies that looked at autism and other a-spec identities such as aromanticism.

My interviewees were themselves aware of this correlation: JK, for example, said that xyr autism "just adds [a] layer to my experience as an a-spec person especially knowing that there are a solid amount of autistic asexual people," and a number of the other people I spoke to explicitly acknowledged a connection between their autism and neurodiversity more generally – their unique way of looking at and being in the world – and their experiences of sexuality and romantic attraction.

DC for example said:

> ADHD and autism mean that I've never really had the social standard experience of interpersonal relationships, but I didn't find out about them until after I'd found out that I was a-spec so it's hard to define them in terms of each other. I guess it's just one more thing that's assumed to be part of the normal human experience that I just don't grok.

While HI said (my emphasis):

> ...autism affects how I observe, think and socialise, making it

> the most dominant feature I have. It plays a huge part in how I identify. Seeing the world through logical and literal terms, it somewhat filters out the things that don't make sense, like certain social norms and rules. That I'm asexual might be due to my minimal need for intimacy and minor need to have a relationship just to not be alone. In some ways, if asexual was instead *autisexual*, then maybe I'd rather identify with that more, but as it is, there is no such identity and therefore asexual and demisexual is as close as I get to what is my identity in regards to sexual attractions.

My interviewees' accounts suggest that, rather than one identity "causing" the other, both these ways of being are instead characterised by a willingness, or even a need, to discard restrictive social norms and expectations, especially those as pervasive and rigid as the norms surrounding sexuality and gender. BH said, when asked about the interaction between her asexuality and being autistic:

> I don't think it directly impacts my identity, but I think being neurodiverse means that I'm less willing to act in the way society expects because society expects it. I think if I were neurotypical, I might be more willing to date men and settle into a long-term relationship because I'm not completely against either thing, and that's certainly the social norm for a Mennonite woman in her twenties.

When asked to describe her gender, HI mentioned:

> Being autistic, social norms that are gendered are just illogical to me and in short I simply didn't care about these rules. I see my body as a mere vessel where my mind is inhabited. I could've

> been anyone and it wouldn't have mattered to me. Because of this, I find autigender and agender much more accurate for my perception of myself.

HI's use of the word "autigender" puts into words that connection between being autistic and disregarding social norms that, for allistic people, may seem like organic, essential parts of being a person, in the same way sexual or romantic attraction might seem universal and all-encompassing to an allo person.

Sensitivity to touch, too, may be another experience that autistic and specifically sex-repulsed asexual people have in common. DC mentioned a discomfort with physical contact from anyone other than her current partner, and the way this influences her experiences of sexuality and attraction:

> ... he falls into a very small category of people with whom I feel safe enough to have intimate physical contact, and since all intimate physical contact between "lying together on the sofa watching a film" and "penetrative sex" kind of falls within the same general category for me, it doesn't make much difference to me what variety of sensual intimacy we practise.

DC's words about intimacy and feeling, as she puts it, "less vigilant about sensory input" around certain people, resonate with the experiences of a number of the people I spoke to who were sex repulsed. For example, BC describes themself as becoming "completely sensorily overwhelmed" during sex.

One of the most fundamental commonalities, however, may simply be the liberatory feeling of finding the right words to describe your experience: in an interview on the *What the Trans* podcast, Felix, an autistic nonbinary person, described how they felt when they received their diagnosis: "Yeah, a big sense of self-acceptance and self-understanding... I was able to understand myself better and love myself more." Jo Ross-Barrett, the other autistic nonbinary interviewee (who is also asexual), said that a "lack of interest in and awareness of other people's opinions was a major benefit of being autistic...[it] led me to focus on what's authentic for me." HI says of her autism:

> If anything, having the label and condition makes it easier to understand why I'm not like others and it hasn't made my relationship difficult. I think having the labels have made it easier to clearly communicate our needs in the relationship.

Throughout this part of the book, I've been looking at what different intersections of identity have to teach us about the complexities of being a-spec, and about sexuality and romantic attraction overall.

There are forces acting on all of us that are beyond our control. And it's impossible to fully explore the extent to which all of us are compromised, denied self-knowledge – as a-spec, but also as people of colour, as disabled people, as women, as men, as queer – by the rigid social norms and expectations that have been created to maintain the status quo.

There is a whole swathe of communities who have been pathologised, punished because of the biomedical community's vested interest in categorising people and policing our sexualities.

The forces, institutions, norms, expectations that tell us we are bad because we are different are the same ones that pit us against each other.

This means that the political project of a-spec liberation cannot take place in a vacuum. And an a-spec community that doesn't seek cooperation, solidarity and community across identity boundaries cannot lead to our liberation.

Discussion questions

1. If you consider yourself to be disabled, neurodiverse or mentally ill, how do you think (if it does at all) your disability, neurodivergence or mental illness interacts with your experience of attraction, romance and sexuality?
2. Do you find other people have certain expectations or preconceived ideas about you, to do with sexual or romantic performance, based on the fact that you are disabled, neurodiverse or mentally ill?
3. Try to think about your own preconceived notions about disabled, neurodiverse, or mentally ill people. Is there a sexual or romantic dimension to these attitudes? If so, try to interrogate what it is and where it came from.

Friends and Family

A few years ago, I made the conscious decision to cultivate my friendships. My career was gathering speed and I was constantly snowed under with work, and it occurred to me that if I didn't put effort into them, it would be all too easy for the relationships I valued most to simply slip away. Moving to Scotland from the US made me realise how easy it was to lose touch with people, even those I cared about, and I didn't want it to happen again. On the other hand, with limited time to socialise – limited still further by the pandemic – I didn't want to spend it with people who didn't nourish me.

So I had to start deciding who I wanted to keep in my life. I had never had this opportunity before: for the first time in my life I was living away from home and not at school, so my friends were no longer simply the people I saw every day. After a few years in Edinburgh, I did have co-workers and flatmates that I considered friends because we saw each other a lot, but I also knew enough people now that I could pick and choose who to spend my time with. I was gratified to find that there were some genuinely good people I wanted to keep in my life – and they seemed to want to keep me around too.

I also started to realise that, as my friends and I were ageing and growing, we were also more and more *coupled up*. I had the sudden realisation that there would always be a risk (especially as, at that time, I didn't see a long-term relationship on the horizon for me) that the people I loved would give up what we had in favour of romantic-sexual partners or growing families.

I agonised over this a lot; back in my mid-twenties, a friend getting into a relationship could be enough to send me into a spiral of depression and anxiety, simultaneously worried I'd lose the friend and reminded that (as I thought then) I'd be forever alone.

Nowadays I'm a lot less insecure. I have a network of people I value and who value me, many of whom are in couples or who want relationships but who still put in the work of maintaining our friendship. I've also realised recently that I've managed, through coincidence or unconscious effort, to build friendships with other a-spec people, many of whom I didn't know were on the ace spectrum until I started writing this book.

These friendships are what we need them to be, and again, for the first time in my life, I've been able to actively shape the most important relationships in my life. My best friend is a trainee therapist. Like me, after some heavy setbacks like moving countries and losing time to mental and physical illness, they're back on track, working hard to build their career. We initially bonded over working on a group project where we were the only two who did any work. So a huge part of our friendship right now is an understanding that both of us are regularly going to be busting our asses, and that free time will be limited. So after spending a huge amount of time together, relying on each other, during the pandemic, nowadays we see each other when we can – a walk here, a trip to the public pool there. We consciously try not to take more than the other person can give, each allowing the other to step back if they're stressed or exhausted. That's what the best friendships are to me: a bond flexible enough for both parties to get what they need, and strong enough to endure absence and hardship.

I knew I was going to talk about relationships when I started writing this book, but I didn't want to do what I'd seen in so much other writing on a-spec issues, which was to centre sex and romance despite the fact that, for so many of us, sex and romance are the least important forces in our lives. I didn't want to talk about what a-spec people *didn't* want, or *don't* feel. Instead, I wanted to focus positively on what we *do* care about, the relationships that mean the most to us. I asked the people who shared their experiences with me to describe the most important relationships in their lives:

> They aren't in your life by accident. They choose to be there. Every day. And you choose them in return. EP

> I feel like I need the warmth that they transmit to me. JTS

> ...the closest thing I've experienced to "true love"... EF

> ...with you always, even when all of the other relationships fall apart. AK

> Strong relationships that I will commit to for life. VC

> I can be myself without prejudice. HI

> ...my relationships with them are all different. They are all fulfilling in different ways. AQ

> Human connection makes life worth living. NT

These were only the most poetic answers – there were many more with a similar sentiment. Out of the nearly 40 people I spoke to in depth, only four didn't list "friends" or "friendships" in the answer to this question.

When asked why these relationships were so important, most of the answers centred around trust, commitment and reliability: the people you could count on to support you and make you feel safe. As OP put it, "We can share our hurt together, and our traumas, and we can be there for each other when that happens..."

The people I spoke to deeply valued bonds with people we could feel comfortable enough around to be ourselves, mutually free of judgement. For someone of a marginalised and often invisible orientation, it's doubly important to invest our time and energy in people who we know won't judge us or try to change us.

Just as I'll explore later on when I discuss familial relationships and coming out, an allo friend or loved one's *personal* stake in sexuality and relationships, in the maintenance of amatonormativity, can put a strain on their relationship with us and create conflict that in fact has nothing to do with our aromanticism or asexuality, and everything to do with how the other person *feels* about it.

This is part of why friendships are so important to so many of us: at its healthiest, friendship is an unconditional type of love, free from obligation and never transactional. A friendship ensures that everyone involved can maintain boundaries, getting and giving what each of us needs emotionally, especially where a romantic or sexual relationship might leave us feeling like we owe the other person something we're not able to give.

LH, who is grey-asexual, described a long-standing friendship, explicitly *sexual*, that she'd been in before she realised she was grey-ace:

> Funnily enough, one of my longest relationships was only sexual in nature, a "friends-with-benefits" arrangement. The fact that I was able to choose when to solicit that friend and turn him down the rest of the time, while trusting he could go to other people if his sex life with me was "not enough", was a great source of comfort for me. He was a more experienced man who had offered to teach me the "basics of sex" without any pressure or any ties (sounds terrible when you phrase it like that, but I was horribly self-conscious of my lack of experience back then and very grateful to be able to go to a friend).

While LH's case isn't typical, it does demonstrate the way friendships become places of safety, free of obligation. LH was able to get what she needed at the time, in a safe and judgement-free environment, "no strings attached".

This is because the word "friendship" itself is capacious: it's not exactly a category you can draw a strict boundary around. Compared to romance and sexual desire, there's far less cultural baggage around what friendship should feel like or look like, and this allows us to create it from the ground up each time. This unconditionality and freedom from rigid expectations means that friendship can be anything we want it to be, and the importance of this flexibility cannot be overstated.

This is often in sharp contrast, then, to our relationships with blood family. As countless queers throughout the centuries have discovered, immediate family bonds – fraught with the expectations of reproduction and family-building, and the tension of being close to someone you haven't *chosen* to have in your life – can be volatile, brittle or toxic.

Despite the delicacy of these bonds, though, the second most popular answer to the "important relationships" question, mentioned by 18 out of 39 people, was "family", especially immediate family such as parents. FG sums up this tension when she says, "as much as it bothers me that I have to stay closeted, my most important relationships are with my parents".

Our blood relatives are often the people who know us best, or at least who've known us the longest, and seen us grow and change over the years; the close bonds we have with them can be as stifling as they are strong. Our families have a huge influence over our own ideas about family and the shape our intimate relationships take: parents and relatives are often the most powerful enforcers of social and cultural values, especially when it comes to domestic matters. Parents and grandparents especially have a "stake" in whether or not we pair up, start families of our own and have children.

I'm probably very lucky, then, that my parents have never pressured me to find a partner or get into a romantic relationship. In high school, at an age when most of my friends were pairing up and exploring their sexuality, my parents were probably relieved I seemed to show no interest. Even at university, when I entered my first romantic relationship, they were supportive but hardly ecstatic.

This may have something to do with my parents' own experiences with intimate relationships. My parents split up when I was in my early teens, and like all divorces, it wasn't always pretty. I watched – though as a teenager I hardly paid much attention – as my parents' affection for each other withered. After the divorce, I heard a lot about relationship strife as my dad dated and broke up with a series of girlfriends, while my mom remained – and remains to this day – happily single. So I've come to realise that this time in my life, by all accounts during my formative years, probably had a huge effect on my own attitudes towards romantic partnerships, instilling a reluctance to enter them willy-nilly, a caution around them that is more or less healthy depending on how you look at it. Any illusions I might have had about love transcending all, or about romantic partnership being the most pure and enduring, were probably stripped away around this time, and I came to see friendships as the more reliable, sustainable source of companionship, support and intimacy.

This journey is paralleled in a somewhat more extreme way by BC, who is demisexual: when asked whether they experience romantic attraction, BC says, "Yes, though because my parents are in an emotionally abusive relationship, I'm a little wary of feeling romantic unless there's already an emotional connection I can trust."

There's so much history and baggage shared between family members that judgement can easily become clouded. Unlike our friends, our parents and other older relatives are not disinterested observers when it comes to sexuality and relationships: the way we choose to live our lives can take on extra layers of meaning depending on our shared history, and their wants and expectations for us. It can stir up prejudices, raise fears around legacy and inheritance and continuing the family name. What parents think is best for their children is often heavily coloured by generational or cultural ideas around family and procreation, and questions of obligation – what parents and children might "owe" each other.

Older relatives, especially parents and grandparents, often have a very personal stake in the maintenance of familial networks, and in their children's willingness to produce children of their own. Countless cultures worldwide place high value on having children and grandchildren and rely heavily on the support network of extended family. For some, the idea of a younger relative not having kids is like a tree branch being cut off at the trunk. Ria, the Filipino AceCon panellist, described trying to convince her family-driven Filipino parents that she was asexual:

> They would say...eventually you are going to want that support system with you, and by support system they only expect it to be family... You always fall back on family, and if you don't have a family at the end of your life, then there's really no point, in their eyes. And it took so long of fighting my parents for them to accept that I really do want to be independent.

So while a number of us listed immediate family among our most important relationships, the same people often described these relationships as complex, fraught and involving a certain amount of obligation or baggage. HG, for example, says, "My grandma whom I'm closest to doesn't accept me which hurt more than I want to admit."

A parent might say to their a-spec child, "I just want you to be happy," or "I want you to have the happy marriage I didn't have." They might say "I want grandchildren," or "You'll need a spouse and children to take care of you when you get old." Rarely do these sentiments actually, truly, have the a-spec person's best interests in mind. As LG says:

> I've always been awkward around kids, said I've never wanted them *and still* I have the occasional relative who says things like "But it's different when they're yours" or "You'll change your mind when you reach a certain age." Do I have to be childless and unmarried at 40 to be taken seriously?

Many people in fact cited their parents or older relatives among the reasons they felt pressured to hide their a-spec identity. BH, after being forced to move back in with her parents due to the pandemic, said she couldn't be open about her asexuality due to "fear of being kicked out of the house". FG, likewise, says, "I have to make my parents think I'm totally straight, hide anything or lie about its symbology [sic] that is an ace flag reference."

The tension between needing to rely on parents for shelter or even emotional support, while at the same time feeling obliged to hide a part of who we are, was a common theme. It's a long, arduous journey for most of us to fully embrace being a-spec. It takes courage to be vulnerable enough to share it with the people we're close to, and to be rejected for something that's not within our control, a fundamental part of who we are, within a relationship we don't have the option of simply stepping away from, can be intensely difficult, even devastating.

The best friendships, then, are the ones that offer trust, reliability and support, free of cultural or emotional baggage and judgement clouded by social expectations. Our friends are the ones who see us as we are. Friendships can be demanding, they can be sites of conflict where we challenge each other and disagree, but at their best they are unconditional and free from expectations around each other's "lifestyle". And unlike romantic or sexual relationships they come with very few pre-packaged duties or responsibilities. Instead, they are flexible, mutually negotiated and robust because of this.

For a great number of queer people, close friendships take on the role of found family, providing support and positive regard where biological family have failed to deliver. Maybe predictably, many people said they actively tried to prioritise friendships with other queer people, a-spec or allo, for exactly this reason.

Many of these friendships were online, with many people also acknowledging the difficulty – especially in non-urban settings – of finding other a-spec or even other queer people in person, especially in locations where it's less safe to be open about that part of yourself. And despite our community's growing visibility, a number of my interviewees expressed with resignation an assumption that they would probably never meet another a-spec person offline. When asked how it felt to know there were other asexual people out there, RK says, "I mean, it's nice. But it's pretty niche. I doubt I'll ever find another ace in real life."

So while online friendships might be considered by some as "less serious" than in-person ones, more tenuous or likely to drift apart, they are also not limited by geographic or time constraints. In the increasingly distanced and globalised world we live in, messaging or video chat allows us to stay in touch on our own terms. And again, perhaps in parallel to the difference between friendships and other intimate relationships, they also lack the structures and expectations of in-person availability that "conventional" offline friendships entail. Indeed, some of my best friends are people with whom I've managed to stay in touch despite one or both of us moving to a different country.

Friendships are committed, mutually nourishing emotional and intellectual bonds. They don't necessarily come with a sexual or romantic obligation, or any kind of obligation at all. At their core, my best friendships are built on care and understanding of each other's needs. I'm allowed to step away from them when I need to, and I can trust that they're robust enough not to wither away before I can tend to them again.

Perhaps because of how valuable close friendships are, there was also an undercurrent of tension or unease to the way the people I spoke to discussed them. Like all relationships, friendship is a two-way street, and a number of people were keenly aware of a precarity associated with being friends with an alloromantic or allosexual person in a world that teaches us to prioritise romance and sex.

This is because, as important as they are to so many people, our society devalues friendships. We've created a hierarchy that enshrines romantic love and sexual connection at the very top, and which consequently places friendships near the bottom. In 2010, blogger IrrationalPoint wrote about the relative importance that society ascribes to the various relationships in a person's life:[1]

> ...from a very young age, we are taught The Relationship Hierarchy. Which is something like: blood ties and marriage ties trump other sorts of ties. Sexual relationships trump non sexual relationships. You have only one partner, who shall be your sexual partner and your lawfully-wedded spouse, and no other partners, and they trump all other relationships. Marriages that produce children trump non-procreating relationships, but Thou Shalt Not Be A Single Parent. "Family" and "Friends" are distinctive sets of people, and "Family" trumps "Friends". "Friends" should mean only people of the same sex, but otherwise, same sex friends trump other-sex friends. You shall be emotionally intimate only with same-sex friends, unless you are a man, and then Thou Shalt Not Have Emotions.[2]

Most of the people I spoke to were acutely aware of the relationship hierarchy, even if they didn't name it as such. When asked if her experience of being a-spec had been shaped or affected by mainstream culture, VC said: "Yes, there is so much pressure and expectations that being in a romantic and/or sexual relationship is what I ultimately want when it really isn't. It upsets me that mainstream culture doesn't value friendships enough."

AB was even more emphatic:

> I think it's important to not compare different types of relationships with one another and create a hierarchy of importance

> (like "romantic relationships are deeper and more meaningful than friendships" etc.) All relationship types can be important and meaningful and it's extremely stigmatising and damaging to overvalue romantic relationships to other types just because they are romantic in nature. I hate nothing more than to lose friends because they started to date and suddenly I became "unimportant" or "not a priority" because the relationship we had was "just" platonic. I care extremely deeply about my friends and these situations break my heart.

A lot of the ways we are taught to talk about friendships contains a tacit assumption that they're the defining relationships of childhood and adolescence, to be gradually phased out as we explore, seek out and settle on a single romantic/sexual partnership. We spend our free time as children and adolescents with friends, and in early adulthood we might live with friends, but it's generally assumed that "when we grow up" we'll end up living with a romantic partner (or, if we're very unlucky, alone).

There's often an assumption within a conventional romantic/sexual relationship that moving in together – meaning in practice that almost all of our time is spent with the romantic partner – is the "next step", and that if we don't do so, the relationship is doomed to fail. The nuclear family is seen as the building block of society, and all the different forces driving us towards it creates a current that is difficult to swim against.

So the position friendships occupy in our adult lives is subject to the same maturity narrative that paints asexual people as immature or "going through a phase", and aromantic people as unfulfilled or as not having "found the right person yet": this narrative defines sex and romance as the end goals of any "serious" or committed relationship, regardless of whether the people involved find those elements desirable or fulfilling.

It's very difficult to disentangle oneself from this maturity narrative, both in our lives as we grow up and within relationships themselves, which are considered to "grow" from something childish like friendship to something mature like romance and sex. (In fact, I've just become aware while typing this that, in having the chapter move from a discussion of friendships to family to romantic and sexual relationships, I might be inadvertently recreating the relationship hierarchy!)

I don't think any of us really make a conscious decision to see relationships this way: it's a received perspective from the media and the narratives we're given as young people, and it's shaped by the social scripts we're given by our families and cultural or religious communities. We are taught that once a relationship has become very close, it becomes "something more", and *ceases to be* a friendship. Even the phrase "something more" is telling: it's a value statement that explicitly positions friendships as "less": once a friendship reaches a certain level of intensity, intimacy or closeness, it "evolves" into a romantic relationship, a different beast entirely.

A number of my interviewees expressed not only an awareness of the way friendships are devalued but also fears like those I experienced as my friends and I hit our mid-twenties and early thirties, around what ageing would mean for the most important relationships in their lives. The idea that, once they all reached a certain age, their allo friends would set aside their childish things, settling down with romantic partners and no longer needing or wanting to put energy into the friendships that the a-spec person prized so highly. Furthermore, there was an idea that the allo person in the friendship might see no problem with this reallocation of time and energy: society tells us at every turn that romance and sex are to be prized, prioritised and sought after, and that once you had those things you were successful and didn't need anything else.

AQ put it in stark terms:

> I sometimes feel like since I can't experience romantic and/or sexual attraction, I'll be alone forever, especially when all my friends move on and start getting married and having kids. I also hate the fact that I feel like my friends are according less attention and care on our friendship than they do their romantic relationships. Sometimes it just makes me [feel] worthless.

When asked what friends or family can do to support her as an aroace person, BH advocated for clarity and communication – a theme that would crop up over and over again as I worked on this section of the book – and attention to the needs of all parties:

> Friends in particular should be really clear about what our relationship means to them because I often feel like I'm more invested in friendships than the other person... Being a-spec can be really isolating, particularly now that I'm at an age at which most of my friends are in serious relationships. At first, I struggled a lot with feeling broken, as if my identity was a failure of some kind, but now I struggle more with anxiety about the future and finding a partner/family/community outside of a traditional marriage.

Overall, almost a third of the people I spoke to in depth expressed worries along these lines. Some, like LM, saw things in a slightly more positive light: "More of my friends are getting married or have partners than they did when I was younger, like my best friend just bought a house with her boyfriend. I'm feeling that difference more, but I'm still comfortable in who I am." When asked what their friends could do to support them, they said:

> I really appreciate it when they don't neglect our friendship after getting partners. When my best friend got a boyfriend, I thought I'd end up being lower priority and she'd be spending all her time with him. Instead, we're both key parts of her life, and our relationship is probably closer now than it was before. Another close friend, even after he moved in with his partner he didn't decrease the amount of time he spent with me, or make me feel left out for not having a partner.

Rather than neglect their friendships with them, LM's allo friends made an effort to resist the considerable social pressure to prioritise their romantic partnerships. Thanks to this work on their part, their friendships with LM were enriched or deepened, rather than spread thin as one might expect. Making the extra effort *not* to neglect a friendship means extending a very specific type of care, care that a-spec people often value deeply.

A number of us, myself included, have been sowing seeds for our future by nurturing friendships with other a-spec people. JH said, "these two [the other a-spec people she knows] are two of my closest friends right now. Possibly this is not a coincidence, and more of my friends find themselves in partnerships that demand most of their time. Or maybe that's just correlation..." and when discussing the important relationships in her life, "a lot of the struggling I've been doing in coming to terms with my asexual identity comes down to the place of significant relationships in my life and whether those relationships can be lasting or deepen".

This sowing of seeds doesn't always happen on purpose – sometimes the people we're drawn to have "ace vibes", or just seem to have similar priorities to us about the things that matter in life. Over the last year or so, I've come to realise that a significant number of my closest friends are actually a-spec themselves. At a small Halloween party this year I threw with a friend, I suddenly broke off in the middle of a sentence, having had the happy realisation that all the people I had invited, who were now all chatting and getting to know each other, were members of the a-spec community. So while I still have some anxieties around what I'll do when I grow older, if I'm not in a committed partnership, I no longer fear I'll be completely alone.

A cynical interpretation of the maturity narrative that still shapes so much of how we engage with relationships might dictate that, as we reach sexual maturity, the biological urge to procreate and build families shades out other forms of human connection. But in the same way that we as humans are working towards overcoming our natural fear of outsiders and the unknown, or our instinct to consider nature and nonhuman life from a utilitarian perspective, working to set aside these instincts also offers huge potential benefit.

Popular culture abounds with stories of people in committed romantic/sexual partnerships who stray, having affairs because they're dissatisfied or feeling that something is "missing" from the (singular) important relationship in their life. To an a-spec person, the solution might seem obvious: no one person can give you everything you need, and expecting them to do so – and for them to expect the same of you – is a recipe for disaster.

It takes a lot of hard work to maintain friendships, to care for more than one or two other people in your life, and not everyone has the stamina or the willingness to spend that time or energy. But the benefits, the robust network you can build, full of people you can go to when you're not getting something you need, are worth it. Because the thing about friendships is that they're sites of mutual care: a network of friendships is like a garden, full of variety and therefore more healthy, robust and sustainable than a single crop. And like a vegetable garden, if you put work and energy into it, it will nourish you in return.

Discussion questions

1. Think about the non-romantic/non-sexual relationships in your life. What do you get from these relationships? How do they nourish you? What do you bring to them? How important are they to you, and has this importance changed over time?
2. Think about the friendships in your life. What do you "get from" each of these people that you don't get anywhere else? What do you give them? Do these relationships feel transactional or obligational in any way?
3. Think about the ways in which your relationships with each of your close friends differs from the others.
4. Can you think of a time when a friend prioritised a romantic partner over their relationship with you? How did it make you feel?

What Is Love?

The languages of the world are rife with "untranslateable" words or phrases, used to describe different types of love or nuances of human connection. The concept of *gezelligheid* is very important in Dutch culture, describing a feeling of comfortable togetherness with loved ones that is hard to sum up.[1] In Japanese, 甘え, or *amae*, specifically refers to a type of desire to be taken care of, that can describe the relationship between a person and their boss, spouse, parent or teacher.[2] The Turkish word ciğerpare, or "liver-part", refers to someone – equally relevant to a lover or a friend – who is so close to you as to be like a part of your own body,[3] something like the English phrase "ride or die".

A number of these words and phrases relate specifically to romantic love and allow for a bit more nuance than is readily available in English. Japanese has a term, 恋の予感, *koi no yokan*, that resembles the English phrase "love at first sight", but goes farther than English, acknowledging the quixotic nature of falling for someone you hardly know – that first impressions are not always the best foundation for a lasting relationship.[4] French and Romanian both have idiomatic expressions acknowledging that love is not always mutual or requited, that it does not always transcend all, and that this lack or failure of connection is as much a part of human relationships as the "happily ever after" that we see in films.[5]

Some of these words – such as Urdu *naz*, ناز, the pride and confidence of being the object of another person's love or desire[6] – express reflexivity, how attractive *attraction itself* can be, in a way that reminds me of the a-spec term *reciprosexual*. Others such as Russian однолюб, *odnoliub*,[7] a person who only has one great love in their life, or who is only capable of loving one person at a time, seem to describe something that likewise isn't admitted by conventional ways we talk about relationships in English.

The ancient Greeks famously acknowledged the existence of a number of different types of love,[8] categories whose definitions and connotations changed over time. More than one of these types of love and affection could exist simultaneously in the same person. Words like *pragma*, a kind of long-term commitment and care that comes from knowing another person intimately, or *philia*, the love between close friends, acknowledge that sexual-romantic bonds are not the only way for two people to love each other.

Framing these different types of affection and passion as all equally important, too, suggests an understanding that no single person in your life can fulfil all of your needs. And while it's hard to know how actual people in ancient Greece used these words, their existence nonetheless evokes a time and place where deep, lasting and intimate bonds that were neither sexual nor romantic could still have been celebrated and respected.

By bringing up these words, I'm not necessarily saying that speakers of the languages I mentioned above are more enlightened about relationships than English speakers, or that your native language lacking a word for something means you're incapable of understanding it. Instead, I'm trying to explore the spaces between the words we're given in English, the wiggle room where other ways of being – that don't centre around sexual and romantic attraction – can be acknowledged.

Those of us with non-normative identities often have to find ways to talk about the relationships we make for ourselves, using tools that are often unequal to the task. I recently grappled with this problem personally, in a group chat about a film night I was planning with some friends. I wanted to ask if I could invite the person I was dating but didn't know how to refer to her. She wasn't quite a girlfriend or a partner at this point – we hadn't been seeing each other for long enough. But we'd met on a dating app, so it felt weird to just call her "my friend". "Is it okay if I invite my...friendperson?" I texted the group, "My personfriend?"

A major theme so far in this book has been that, in many cases, the language we are *given* to talk about sex, romance and ways of loving in general is totally inadequate; this is why the a-spec community has collaboratively built a better vocabulary for describing our lived experience.

But ace-spectrum people are not the only ones who have had to express a deep, passionate bond using language that isn't up to scratch. Literature and history are awash with tales of "great loves" that can only inadequately be described by conventional language. Take the writer Iris Murdoch and philosopher Philippa Foot: the pair had a well-documented, passionate friendship, which Sukaina Hirji and Meena Krishnamurthy discussed in a *New Statesman* article entitled "What is romantic friendship?"[9]

While Murdoch and Foot's relationship wasn't necessarily sexual – according to Hirji and Krishnamurthy, it became sexual at one point before the pair decided that "their feelings for each other were not best expressed in this way" – but it nonetheless seemed to involve commitment, intimacy and deep feeling.

Hirji and Krishnamurthy write, "part of what Murdoch describes...is an inability to really understand what she feels, or what she needs from Foot..." Without the simultaneously guiding and limiting structures of social norms – both women married and had (presumably) romantic-sexual relationships with others outside their friendship – the two women struggled to know how to feel, how to articulate themselves and how to draw boundaries. Murdoch wrote, "Sometimes I feel I have to invent a language to talk to you in, though my heart is very full of definite things to say."[10]

As tempting as it is, I think it's something of a fool's errand to try to ascribe current-day identities to even very recent historical figures – for example, to speculate about whether Murdoch or Foot might have been on the asexual spectrum. Identity labels are more than just accurate descriptions of the way a person feels: they are tied as much to a person's current social and political context as they are to how that person experiences attraction.

And of course, it's almost impossible to determine, without being able to ask them, how someone *really* experiences something as nebulous as attraction or desire – *especially* given the absence of adequate language to describe it. The language the a-spec community is using was developed mostly over the last few decades: so most people for the wide span of history, of course, haven't had access to anything like it.

Nonetheless, there's something that resonates with me in the sentiments expressed by Murdoch, her bewilderment and frustration at the way the language we're given seems to try to force us to call ourselves and our relationships one thing or another, neither word quite right. It's a frustration, an exasperated confusion, that *feels* very a-spec to me.

But relationships such as Murdoch and Foot's romantic friendship did not always exist in isolation, either: there have actually been times in the Anglophone West where the ambiguity between friendship and romance has been acknowledged, even accepted. "Boston marriages" were a type of Victorian-era relationship where middle- and upper-class women, especially at American women's colleges, would live together in a committed, romantic, but "not necessarily sexual" relationship.[11]

Boston marriages were well-documented at the time, and widely acknowledged to exist within their cultural context. They weren't taboo, necessarily, but they were new, and unconventional, and therefore notable. Women in the separate, self-contained communities of women's colleges could build, for perhaps the first time in American history, lives for themselves outside the roles that had historically been ascribed to them. Women in these relationships didn't need to shape their lives around finding husbands and building nuclear families.

It's likely that many Boston marriages *were* sexual: after all, most of the population of the earth is sexual, and sex is one of many ways we express our feelings for the people we love. But despite the fact that society likes to elevate sex, drawing a line around it to keep it separate from everything else, I see no reason why sexual and non-sexual Boston marriages should be considered fundamentally different. The thing that unites these relationships is the way the people in them actively shaped them in spite of prevailing social norms and expectations.

Regardless of whether they were homo*sexual* or even homo*romantic*, Boston marriages were unequivocally *queer*: in their own time they subverted traditional gender roles and social expectations. By building these relationships for themselves, women were exercising agency over the shape of their lives that had for most of history been denied them – the same thing that a-spec people in queerplatonic partnerships are doing today. These romantic friendships involved a carving out of space: the radical, queer act of embracing rather than pushing away one's feelings for another person, even if they don't fit the conventional narrative.

Split attraction

The philosopher Carrie Jenkins wrote[12] about the changing way our society is hierarchising sex, romance and friendship. She argues that romantic love is both biologically and socially constructed, and that the social "script" we've been given – of finding your soulmate, settling into a lifelong monogamous relationship and having children – is "too narrow to capture the sorts of romantic relationships that many of us find most fulfilling".[13]

And it *does* seem like the idea of the nuclear family as the building block of society – the foundation on which amatonormativity has been built – is beginning to crumble. As the shape of the world changes around us – our movements increasingly global, our workplaces increasingly decentralised, our relationships no longer centred around a family home – and our understandings of sexuality and gender change as well, it's clear we need to complexify our thinking around relationships.

Part of the efforts to do just this has led to the creation of something called the split attraction model (or SAM).[14] The SAM is a way of deliberately de-coupling sex and romance. Within the SAM, a person is seen as having both a sexual and romantic orientation. While connected, these don't necessarily go hand in hand. A person can be asexual but alloromantic, bi- homo- or heterosexual but demiromantic, pansexual and aromantic, and so on.

The split attraction model is the reason I am able to call myself asexual and grey-aromantic – and my interviewees generally articulated their orientations in ways that took split attraction as a given. Within the a-spec community, the SAM is very much common knowledge.

The SAM is also the reason I am able to distinguish between the specific marginalisations, and often very different lived experiences, of asexual versus aromantic people, and an understanding of sexuality as separate from romantic orientation was part of my decision to use "a-spec" instead of just "ace" as an umbrella term.

By disconnecting two things that are usually treated as equivalent and co-occurrent, the SAM allows for a deeper exploration of desire, attraction and intimacy. Obviously, for this reason, it's been widely embraced within the a-spec community, but the concept isn't entirely alien outside it as well: pop culture often speaks of "sexless marriages" and "one-night stands" – neither of these phenomena are ever very far from mainstream consciousness. But the key difference here is that sexless marriages and one-night stands are often associated with unhappiness, unhealthiness, lack or dysfunction. At the very least, they're usually discussed in a context of something "missing".

RH, when asked if there was pressure to hide her identity as demiromantic, was explicitly aware of this negative connotation: "I still feel a certain level of shame because of society and media's idea of what people who have sex without romance are like, as well as well-meaning friends who didn't understand my experience, and so said insensitive things."

The language of "something missing" and "dysfunction" strikes a familiar chord with me, reminding me of the way that asexuality has for so long been defined entirely in terms of pathology and lack. By talking about a disconnect between sex and romance in terms of a *missing* physical or emotional connection, an allonormative idea of split attraction can actually contribute to aphobia – for example in RH's words, "society and media's [negative] idea of what people who have sex without romance are like" – the idea that a person who experiences one without the other is ill or unfulfilled in some way.

What the split attraction model *as a model* does, then, is reclaim the idea that sex and romance can exist separately and, further, that there's nothing wrong with this. It legitimises that disconnect by bringing it into the regular (albeit queer) discourse around relationships, attraction and orientation.

The SAM isn't without its critics, even within the a-spec community. For one thing, just like the allonormative categories of gay, straight and bi, it fails to question *why* we have categories in the first place, and therefore its applicability to the messiness of real life is still limited. IJ, who is both ace and nonbinary, articulated these criticisms when discussing their experience of belonging to multiple communities within the LGBTQ+ umbrella:

> I also don't feel like using the split attraction model is necessarily that useful as it feels like you then have to be really specific about your labels, rather than your lived experience or how you might feel and interact with the world. As I mentioned previously, if I was trying to dissect then probably I would be thinking of something like panromantic, but I don't feel like the label is useful.
>
> I did previously consider "lesbian" but found that didn't work for me either in terms of my gender, because though there are many nonbinary lesbians I wouldn't say that's how I feel I interact with the world, and also because I don't know who I could hypothetically be in a relationship with, but I doubt that would be limited to women in this hypothetical circumstance.

IJ's words raise the question, once again, of whether labels are always useful or helpful – what good is the word "red" if the colour I see and the colour you see are completely different? Part of the shortcomings of the split attraction model is that it only goes as far as separating sex and romance – it doesn't help us to understand either term any better. And this is important, because one of the most common answers I got when I asked people if they experienced romantic attraction was "I don't know".

While a number of my interviewees were themselves in intimate relationships with other people, some of them even explicitly romantic-sexual, most were unable to draw a clear dividing line between different, nonsexual types of love or attraction, especially platonic and romantic. If friendships are conventionally thought of as less passionate or committed than romantic relationships, but friendships are the most important relationships in your life, how do you distinguish them from romances? If romantic partners are supposed to be the people we settle down with, but you share a home, domestic tasks and physical affection with a close friend, what's the difference? When it comes to romance, we're told, "You'll know it when you see it." Which is fine, unless, of course, you don't.

Most of the people I spoke to, and I myself, found themselves confused over what, exactly, romantic attraction – "falling in love" – was supposed to feel like. LG, who struggled specifically to come to terms with the aro part of their aroace identity, says:

> It's hard to quantify romantic feelings when you're not sure how they're supposed to feel and if something is romantic or just temporary infatuation or just me just misinterpreting my own feelings?... And if they really are romantic feelings, do they count if they fizzle out really quickly? Or if they exist only when

> things are theoretical and not actually happening? Isn't that amatonormativity at play?

I remember jokingly complaining to my aroace friend, DL, that romance and all its trappings was just a big hoax, a joke at our expense. Many of my interviewees echoed this frustration: DC, when asked what it was like to discover that a-spec identities were a "thing", said: "It was less 'there are other people like me out there' and more 'wait, most of the people out there *aren't* like me and actually literally mean it when they talk about finding people attractive rather than it being, like, conversational shorthand or narrative convention'".[15]

While EL told me, "In middle school I made up crushes to tell my friends about because nobody took 'no one' as an actual answer."

JK, when asked if xe had ever felt romantically attracted to another person, said, "Eh...maybe? It's weird, I have a hard time pulling it apart from sensual attraction so... I tend to lean towards the latter more than romantic impulses." LM, when asked if they'd been in a romantic relationship before, said, "I think I'd like to be in a romantic relationship, but I'm not sure because I've never been in one."

LG, who is grey aroace, describes their experiences of romantic attraction:

> God honestly it's so random. I thought it was only with people I felt close to, but it's not?? I can never predict it. I've had crushes on people for superficial reasons and there's a couple crushes I had on friends were [sic] because I really admired and felt close to them, but that only happened in my teen years. Not sure how much of it was fuelled by hormones. Now that I'm an adult my

crushes have been super light and I lose interest super easy. Which is why I don't bother to do anything with them.

I actually found LG's words refreshing: while they might occasionally feel romantically attracted to someone, romance was not an all-consuming driving force in their life. JK describes a similar experience, almost a type of freedom, from the many conventional expectations around dating and relationships: "[I] found that without any romantic goals for my life that maybe I didn't need to structure my life around finding a romantic partner."

When I asked EL if she had ever been in a romantic or sexual relationship before, she said no, but described her relationship with her best friend, which was sometimes perceived that way by others: "We don't consider our relationship to be romantic and it is not sexual." I was struck by EL's phrasing. When it came to describing the (non)sexual nature of the relationship, there was no doubt or room for negotiation: "It is not sexual." But when it came to romance, the answer seemed to be based less in an objective reality outside EL and her best friend, but instead actively negotiated between them; EL and her best friend do not *consider* their relationship to be romantic, but there is an implication that another two people in a similar situation might consider things a different way.

So, any attempts to define "romance" as separate from sex might already be dead in the water. Over and over, the people I spoke to told me they found it nebulous and hard to quantify. Instead, what seems more useful to me is thinking more deeply about intimacy, and what it means to be close with someone you care about. What do love, affection and intimacy mean when you can't fall back on sex to make their presence clear? What might a committed, loving relationship look like between two people who are not romantically attracted to each other? How can I articulate what I need from my partner if our relationship doesn't look like the couples on TV? And more broadly, what would all of our relationship dynamics look like if we stripped away the behaviours, gestures and arrangements that society expects from us, and instead did whatever felt most intuitive or natural?

It wasn't until I started writing this section of the book that I started questioning what intimacy actually means to me, and, further, what it *could* mean. Something I've come to realise, that I hadn't really seen put into words before – besides a short-lived trend of talking about "love languages" on social media in the late 2010s – is that there *is* more than one kind of intimacy, and it's natural for different people to want, and need, different things from a relationship.

In their essay "Radical Identity Politics",[16] Erica Chu points out that one of the reasons ace-spectrum people are marginalised is because of the way our society thinks about sexuality and attraction, and more specifically the ways that we put people into categories based on that understanding.

The current system uses what Chu calls "sexual object choice" to put people in boxes: if you're attracted to people of the same gender as you, you're gay, if you're attracted to people of the opposite gender, you're straight, and if you're attracted to all genders, you're bi. "Sexual(/romantic) object choice" – orientation – has emerged as the way by which "legitimate" categories of existence are created: who you form romantic and sexual bonds with is seen as a defining feature of who you are.

Like nonbinary folks within binary gender, a-spec people exist outside of those accepted categories, and therefore our existence challenges the validity of that system. Apart from a few times when asexuals have managed to plant their flag alongside bisexuals as another "neither one nor the other" identity, for the most part this system excludes anyone who *has no* sexual-romantic object choice. Essentially, being a-spec means "opting out" of a system that's existed for thousands of years. And just as nonbinary people have to fight for their right to take up space in binary-gendered society, a-spec people often have to work hard to convince others that our ways of being are legitimate.

Chu wonders instead what would happen if we were to break down "what we commonly think of as 'sexuality'" further, or in a different way. Chu suggests a new framework, by which we might consider a person's orientation towards not just the gender of a sexual partner, but also towards partnered sex or any sexual activity at all, or how one feels about non-sexual aspects of a relationship, such as one's orientation towards romantic partners, sensuality, or intimacy. (Note: my definition of "intimacy" is slightly different from Chu's.)[17]

What if the way we categorised people was based around not sexual orientation but orientation towards sex with partners? Under a system where people were grouped based on *whether* they sought out partnered sex – regardless of that partner's gender – "asexual" would be considered a legitimate category. In a world where we labelled people based on orientation towards intimacy, people who didn't desire physical intimacy in any form would be allowed to exist alongside those who do. How would the ways that a-spec people are treated change if we didn't make *attraction to someone* a prerequisite for being counted? How might everyone's perspectives on sex, attraction and desire change?

Like the split attraction model, Chu's model provides a more nuanced way of thinking about desire and attraction and opens up new possibilities for defining relationships and communicating our needs around emotional connection and sexual compatibility.

And Chu's breakdown isn't the only possibilities. I could break intimacy down further and further, making it increasingly granular, but unlike the split attraction model, that's not what I, or Chu, are trying to do. Complex models like Chu's are useful because they let us look at concepts like sex and romance and realise they aren't as rigid, organic and eternal as they might seem. This model is useful not because it creates new boxes to put people in, but because it questions why we have boxes at all. It shows us that there are other possibilities, other ways of expressing care and love – and we owe it to ourselves and each other to explore them.

There are infinite ways to be close to and express love for another person, and it's gradually become clear to me that most of these probably don't fit with the ways we're taught to talk about relationships. Intimacy can be a three-hour conversation in a quiet corner of a pub, or giving your partner a massage after a long day at work, or simply being close to each other in companionable silence, in a way you aren't with anyone else.

This revelation – that there is more to what makes two people compatible than just sexual and romantic chemistry – may seem obvious to the more experienced or emotionally intelligent among us, but it was not obvious to me. I grew up thinking that the fact that I didn't seem to connect with other people in one specific way was a giant problem – a problem so glaring that it seemed to overshadow everything else, despite the fact that I was perfectly capable of being emotionally vulnerable or physically affectionate. These elements of intimacy were always wrapped up so tightly with sex and romance that to separate them, to be able to say *this* is what I want – let alone to get it – seemed like an impossible pipe dream.

So while writing this book, for the first time ever, I've had the opportunity to think deeply about what *I* want in an intimate relationship. To be honest, I've found the process intimidating; I'd become so used to making shift with whatever I was given, even if some of my needs weren't being met.

With this new knowledge, the stakes are higher: now that I've got the language to talk about what I need and want, I owe it to myself, and to my partner, to make those needs known. Communicating about this stuff is still difficult: I still don't quite know how to say what I need to say, and of course, having words for something doesn't necessarily make communicating all that much easier.

Since I've realised I *have* needs and wants within a relationship, outside what is commonly communicated, the responsibility has fallen on me to figure out what those needs are and how to talk about them. What do I find fulfilling in a relationship? What do I enjoy and what could I take or leave? Where are my boundaries?

It also means that, since a relationship is a mutual partnership, I need to be mindful of my partner's needs as well. I can't skate by on the assumption that I will be told what I need to do: I need to seek out this information as part of my care for my partner, precisely *because* I know how hard these things are to talk about.

Another thing I deeply miss about one particular ex, that I'd never had with anyone else before them, was the easy physicality of simply being in our bodies together, of becoming acquainted with each other's bodies in a non-sexual way. We would take baths together, swim, get dressed and undressed at the start or end of a day, without an ounce of embarrassment or shyness, because we trusted and felt safe in each other's presence. If I want that kind of closeness with future partners, especially with asexual or sex-repulsed partners, I'll have to learn to communicate about it carefully.

One of the most fulfilling parts of being in an intimate relationship, for me, is what I've started thinking of as domestic intimacy. Some of my favourite things to do as a couple – and one of the ways being with friends and being with a partner blur together for me – is in cooking together, fixing or building something, or doing a project around the house. Domestic intimacy for me is deeply tied in with the idea of *home*: a place to settle, relax and feel safe with another person or people, which encompasses all the things I mentioned above. There needs to be a reliable connection I can count on, not a fleeting attraction: intimacy with a solid foundation. This is a kind of intimacy I think of as a "requirement" in my relationships – in the same way, I suppose, that an allosexual person might consider "sexual compatibility" as a requirement for theirs.

The people I spoke to also articulated a number of different types of intimacy or closeness that they valued in a relationship. When describing how she knew she was romantically attracted to her current partner, LH says:

> I basically noticed I wanted emotional intimacy and a sensual relationship with her (I'm very physically affectionate). My feelings have matured with time (been together six years) with the increasing conviction that I wanted to form a family unit with her: face life together, be able to rely on each other or share good times together, be there to tell her she's beautiful and see her smile, etc. (Gosh I'm sappy!)

CD said:

> I think of romance as demonstrations of understanding between people – showing each other that they know and understand and care for each other. It may sound silly, but the times I've

> realized that I was attracted to someone romantically usually came when they had made a demonstration like this, even if it was outwardly a small thing – sending me a poem they thought I would like, and their being correct that I would like it; or sending me a magazine clipping because it reminded them of something we'd discussed; or making time to spend with me.

I was struck repeatedly by how it seemed to be the social scripts around dating and relationships, not the reality of our feelings, that shaped how the people I spoke to perceived and spoke about their own relationships.

When asked how she knows she's attracted to someone, LH said (my emphasis):

> I tend to develop crushes on people once I start to know them well and realise I love their personality. The works: I get intimidated by their presence, I look at them with stars in my eyes, I want to kiss them or hold them (no sexual attraction, generally, with maybe a couple of exceptions in my life..., though for reasons mentioned before *I'm now sometimes reinterpreting past "sexual attractions" as my past self forcing that interpretation because that's what I expected to feel, whereas when I think about it I don't think I actually wanted to have sex with these people. The emotional and sensual connection was really what it was about.*) These crushes mostly get demoted to fond friendships over time.

LH is aware of the way compulsory sexuality has shaped her expectations of her own romantic relationships. Her words are interesting because they subvert the conventional narrative of our feelings gradually intensifying from friendship to romantic attraction to sexual attraction over time, though she does still use the language of "demotion" for what could also be described in terms of development or simple transformation, from crush to fond friendship – a change neither positive nor negative.

SKW points out how, once you pull on one thread, the whole messy knot of sexuality and romantic orientation seems to unravel:

> My ability to feel romantic attraction separate from sexual attraction is also one of my reasons for not feeling certain about all the remaining facets of my sexuality, or other forms of attraction; this is due to me (during my early teens, when I thought myself a man) having felt romantic attraction to a close male friend of mine, in spite of not feeling sexual attraction to him (and being quite sure, even at the time, that this wasn't denial due to some kind of internalised homophobia).

So, without the weathervane of sexual attraction pointing us in the right direction, and with romance being so hard to define, the people I spoke to seemed to rely on all sorts of criteria to tell when they're romantically attracted to someone.

Lots of people described just feeling a profound sense of personal attraction, a shift in their way of thinking about the other person. IJ simply describes "thinking of [the other person] in a different way to other people". JTS says, "When I'm constantly thinking about that person and I want to spend a lot of time with him. I feel like I'm weaker when he is around"; and NT puts it, "I know I am romantically attracted when I sincerely desire their company and miss them terribly when they are not around." GH says, "I've spent some time with him and I want to be close to him, get to know him on a more personal level. He's all I think about, and I am happy in my daydreams of him."

SS was one of the few people who was very clear on when and how romantic attraction might emerge:

> I need at least two hours of uninterrupted one-on-one personal conversation, sometimes a lot more, before I might feel anything romantic. If it happens, it'll usually start to develop within the first month of acquaintance. If I've known them for longer than a month and not felt anything romantic, it's probably going to stay as a friendship.

For some people, what romantic attraction looks like might also change, depending on the gender of the person they're attracted to. RR says:

> With men, in the past, I've recognised it pretty early on since I just feel that warm fuzzy "I like this person" feeling. With women, I realised it's been a lot harder for me to realise this. The first time I realised it was actually because I was jealous that my then best friend, now girlfriend, was going to do something entirely platonic, that I regarded as a special thing between us, with another person. I realised pretty quickly after that I was into her.

While EP, when asked what she would look for in a prospective partner, said simply, "Women who intimidate me and men who don't."

> If I like the person enough that kissing them wouldn't be unimaginable. It could be that I'm having such fun with them that I highly enjoy their company, that they are funny, smart and considerate, have interesting topics to talk about, etc. Practically a good friendship can enable a romantic attraction. Intimacy isn't a big part of who I am, so if I want to kiss someone on the lips, then it's a good indicator that I'm romantically attracted. HI [Note: HI uses the word "intimacy" slightly differently to me, to refer specifically to a physical and sensual connection.]

> I want to go on actual dates with the person instead of just hanging out. I might imagine sex with them or not, but mostly I see myself going out to dinner (or well, the equivalent, with COVID out there) with them, kissing, that sort of thing. BC

> As I understand it, if I'm attracted to someone, I want to get to know them better and spend time with them. That sounds like friendship, but I want to spend time with them exclusively, and relax my guard enough to see if they are trustworthy. I generally find I want to cuddle with the person I'm attracted to, a lot. HBJ

> It's hard to tell. It often just happens. Usually, I know something is going on when I try to find excuses to spend some time with the person, or when I do things just to please them. But sometimes it's hard to distinguish romantic attraction from platonic attraction. So if I just don't see myself dating that person, if it's just me wanting them to like me and care for me, it's platonic attraction. If I want to kiss them, it's romantic attraction. LL

On the whole, most of the a-spec people who shared their experiences with me found it difficult to say for certain, "this feeling is romantic, and this is platonic". And while the answers above seem to circle around an implication of exclusivity, time investment and physical touch, few were able to say for certain what distinguished their feelings from friendcrushes or platonic attraction, especially considering that people socialised as female are encouraged to be physically affectionate with their friends.

For many a-spec people, there is no real difference in kind, and not always even in degree or intensity. We can be just as devoted, physically affectionate and emotionally intimate with our friends as we are with a romantic partner. For a lot of us, functionally speaking, there *is* no real distinction between romantic and platonic.

Predictably, a good handful of a-spec neologisms have been created specifically to address or challenge the blurry or even non-existent boundary between romantic and platonic affection. *Alterous* is one of these words, describing relationships or attraction of an in between or ambiguous nature. Alterous attraction is defined as "a form of emotional attraction...not necessarily platonic [or] romantic in nature. For some it may be in between romantic and platonic attraction, and for others it may be completely separate from the romantic/platonic distinction."[18]

When asked if she experiences any kind of attraction for other people, CF says:

> I am not sure about romantic attraction, I am still trying to figure it out. It happened a couple of times that I met people I was very comfortable with, we became very close friends but I realised that I considered them a sort of "special friends". For me it was a little more than friendship, but I had no desire for a romantic relationship with them. That is when I found the term alterous attraction, and it is the word that better defines the kind of feelings I had for those people.

AQ elaborates, noting that different types of connection take longer to form:

> I experience other types of attractions than sexual and/or romantic and I find myself having platonic or alterous crushes (and I might get some romantic crushes in here as well). I guess it kinda depends on time for me to get romantic crushes. Platonic crushes are quicker to set.

Quoiromantic is another word that I had never encountered before beginning this project, and like alterous, I've found it very useful in organising my thinking. LGBTA Wiki defines quoiromantic (also called WTFromantic or whatromantic) as "a term associated with challenging one's own romantic orientation as not personally helpful. It can also include not knowing one's romantic orientation or not wanting to define [it]."[19] In other words, quoiromantic challenges the very idea of "romance" as a useful or distinct category.

As KL, who uses the word *wtfromantic*, said: "I don't think I experience romantic attraction???? But I don't really know what that means??? I like being in a relationship, and my partner is sort of different from my friends but also not????"

For VC, quoiromantic means not being able – or even wanting – to differentiate between one's experience of different types of attraction; it means acknowledging that there's little use in trying to do so. VC says, "It feels less suffocating [than] to try and draw lines between romantic and platonic, by simply acknowledging my love for friends and partners as a nonbinary type of love." VC goes on to say:

> While I can enjoy romantic content in the media, I'm very much romance-confused so I have a complicated relationship with romance and romantic relationships. It's possible that I have experienced romantic attraction before, but I wonder if it was limerence and if other people would've perceived them differently. It's confusing for me to reflect too much on the romantic attraction so I try to focus on the topic of romantic relationships. I don't know which behaviours and activities are romance-coded beyond referring to romance-coded things in the media.
>
> I feel if I were to have a romantic partner I would mostly

> interact with them as I would with very close friends. That elaborates on the identity quoiromantic.

Describing the relationship she has with her friends, VC says: "I experience platonic attraction when I intuitively feel 'good vibes' from new people I meet, but I often feel I fall in love with my friends all over again when we are happy together."

Despite the fact that a conventional allonormative perspective might consider someone who doesn't feel romantically attracted to other people as cold or emotionless, VC's words suggest the opposite: she is full of passion, enthusiasm and commitment towards her friends, the strongest and most fulfilling relationships in her life.

RH, who uses the words demiromantic, quoiromantic and aceflux to refer to herself, describes her experience of attraction as "in between", but still acknowledges that having a word for something doesn't always automatically clear up any confusion:

> I definitely know that I am romantically attracted to my partner, which only came about after we had been in a very close relationship for a while. Before that I would have described my attraction as a very close queerplatonic, in between platonic and romantic. I have been attracted to other people in this in between way before but can't really say for sure that I was romantically attracted to any one of them. I don't really know how I know, sorry!

Neither of these terms are in especially common usage yet. They seem to mainly be used online, spreading quickly within specific close-knit communities like Tumblr, but not necessarily outside them. But what romantic friendships and Boston marriages make clear to me is that something like a-spec relationships, of a kind, have always existed, though always shaped and constrained by their specific context.

Various cultures and communities at various times have created new categories to attempt to articulate the messiness of human connection and the inadequacy of the nuclear family model. Trying to decide for certain whether a relationship is a romance or a friendship may be functionally impossible, a useless exercise, if friendship and romance look different for every single person on earth. But as with romantic friendships and Boston marriages, words like "alterous" and "quoiromantic" are necessary, because the feelings they describe are real.

Discussion questions

1. What does "romance" look like for you? Do you experience romantic attraction? How do you know when you do?
2. Had you heard of the split attraction model before? In what contexts?
3. What does intimacy look like for you? What do you find fulfilling in a relationship, be it romantic, sexual or platonic?
4. How hard or easy do you find it communicating these needs with partners, or even with friends?

Sex

In June of 2021, just in time for Pride season, a hallowed old argument started cropping up again on social media, about whether kink and BDSM paraphernalia should be allowed at Pride marches. One of the arguments made by the conservative "no kink at Pride" side of the conflict was the claim that seeing leather, bondage gear or someone in a puppy play mask constituted a non-consensual sex act, and that these should be banned in order to "protect asexuals". In response, a whole host of asexual people fought back, pointing out that no one actually *in* the asexual community was advocating against kink at Pride, and that, in fact, a-spec people of all descriptions had been part of the kink and BDSM scene for as long as there had been one.[1]

If we were to ban kink at Pride because it meant aces had to "see sexual content" they were uncomfortable with, then we might as well also ban most billboards, bus ads and prime-time TV.

This debate became a flashpoint for looking at larger questions around assimilation and respectability politics in the LGBT+ community. And despite the fact that we had nothing to do with it, aces got drawn into the fight when conservative allos tried to co-opt our asexuality to accomplish their own political aims, in the process revealing that they had fundamentally misunderstood both kink *and* asexuality: assuming that the former is inherently sexual and that the latter is inherently anti-sex.[2]

Despite the fact that *asexual* is the most widely known of all the a-spec identities, plenty of people still readily misinterpret it, assuming that because a person has no interest in having sex with someone else, that they're against sex in all its forms. But despite the fact that asexuality is conventionally defined as not experiencing sexual attraction, the actual attitudes that ace people have about sex *itself* vary hugely from person to person. Among the people I spoke to, there were those who were repulsed by the very idea of sex, there were those who considered it a fun and enjoyable way to connect with a partner and there were those who simply didn't care.

But because sex is highly political and politicised, oftentimes asexuals are cast into the role of "kink shamers", with (often straight, cis) "allies" pitting us against other groups that *they* see as "highly sexual". (Of course, "highly sexual" in these cases usually translates to "queer".) This is all despite the fact that a-spec people know very well what it is to be a sexual minority and have been active in all parts of the queer community for years.

When it comes to thinking about sex, it's important to remember that an asexual person's attitudes towards it are *personal* feelings and opinions – and so are yours. In the same way that a kink or fetish might make you uncomfortable but not actually have any real-world moral or ethical implications, it's important to learn to separate your own personal feelings toward difference from objective reality.

And this parallel to kinks and kinkshaming goes both ways: just because aces as a group might not feel sexual attraction, or be able to empathise with your experience of it, doesn't mean that we're judging you, or trying to assert some sort of moral high ground by "abstaining". An ace person would have to be pretty disconnected from reality to consider an allo person weird, aberrant or otherwise exceptional for being allo. And while it might be tempting for an ace person feeling alienated to conceptualise allos as somehow more dirty, worldly or less "pure", anyone who's experienced marginalisation for being a-spec knows that all of this is just natural human variation; no one way of being is inherently "better" than any other.

From a personal standpoint, I don't really care about sex. The act – and the topic – doesn't excite me, and "sexiness" in another person is an abstract quality at best. Part of what I want to do with this book is to knock sex off its pedestal. Despite what Freud might have us believe, I don't think everything in life is secretly about sex. Sex isn't some kind of "secret language" by which the true meanings of things can be divined, and the act itself often has more to do with ego, insecurity or power than any universal or all-powerful connection between two people.

None of this changes the fact that, in the West at least, sex is nigh-on inescapable. It's a fact of life for most people, allo or ace, and it's been leveraged as a tool to maintain the status quo for thousands of years. This is why it feels so big, universal and important. Sexual preferences and the shape of a person's genitalia (what is conventionally termed their "biological sex") inform the ways we're taught to think about gender, social and familial obligations. Sex permeates advertising and popular culture.

In some ways, it's actually a privilege for me, as an a-spec person, to even be able to say, "I don't care about sex", because for so much of history, sex – like binary gender – has been like water for fish. And because it's so political, with all sorts of cultural meaning ascribed to it, sex has for most of history not been something any of us could choose to "opt out" of, at least

person." And that "that person is sexy" isn't even the same thing as "I want to have sex with that person" either!

Something I noticed early on, which resonated with my own personal experience, was the presence of a heavy cloud of intimidation, even fear, around sex. This seemed to have less to do with a person's repulsion or ambivalence, and more with the way we tend to glorify sex, garlanding it with cultural baggage that makes it seem bigger than it really is. Even among people who had no (or at least didn't mention any) trauma around past sexual encounters, many said they felt, or had in the past felt, fear or intimidation around the idea of having sex. HBJ, for example, said she "really had to work up the courage to try sexual activity. For a long time even kissing was frightening. I don't consider sex to be disgusting, but I did consider it to be scary."

Oftentimes, this intimidation would be directly linked to a lack of access to inclusive sexual education. The feelings of inadequacy and brokenness that emerge when an ace or demi or grey-a person is told that sex is a universal human function can create heavy baggage around the act itself, turning it into simultaneously a shining beacon of human functionality, and a great source of shame. When discussing what would have made coming out as arospec asexual easier, VC, too, echoes this:

> Having decent sex education and education on GRSM (Gender, Romantic and Sexual Minorities)! To be aware from a younger age that not everyone has the same experience and relationship with gender, sex and romance would have allowed me to explore my identity sooner and not feel so out of place.

Even though I've spent the last two years of my life working through all my personal baggage around sex, and coming to understand that having or not having sex is actually not that big a deal, I still often find myself thinking how much easier my life would be, how much less alienated I'd feel from most of my generation's pop culture or casual conversation, if I was just comfortable having casual sex with strangers. The fact that so much of our sex education, and the way we talk about it with young people, assumes everyone *will* experience instant sexual attraction, and in the same way, seems to create a huge mental block around it for those of us who don't.

In terms of their desire to have sex with a partner, Hille *et al.*'s respondents expressed a range of attitudes, from a utilitarian, "I do it because it feels good", to a negotiated willingness contingent on a partner's desire, to a strong disgust or discomfort.

Among the people I spoke to in depth, three groups emerged, though not necessarily equivalent to Hille's. Most of the asexuals I spoke to could be described as either enthusiastic, ambivalent or repulsed (or averse) towards the act of sex. Among those who were sex repulsed, this repulsion could fluctuate over time, or vary both in terms of severity and what it was focused on; for example, a number of people expressed discomfort or disgust for certain aspects of sex or sexuality but not others, like being okay with viewing sexual content but not with being personally sexualised, okay with play above the waist but not below, and so on.

Sex ambivalence

Ambivalence towards sex was one of the most common attitudes I encountered. As KL said, "I'm really comfortable with my sexuality, and I'm not sex averse, so either [having sex with a partner or not] would be fine, but also I find sex not being part of the equation so much more comfortable."

This ambivalence could also manifest as indifference towards *partnered* sex specifically: a trend that I was surprised by but probably shouldn't have been, was the sheer number of people who said that, while they didn't experience sexual attraction for other people, or had no interest in sex with partners, they did still have a libido, and might masturbate when they felt the need. When asked "What's something that a sexual partner does, or can do, to make you feel safe and supported during sex?", NT gave a somewhat tongue-in-cheek answer: "Turn off the lights and try not to interrupt my time with my vibrator by touching me...or speaking...or being in the room with me?"

SKW had some interesting thoughts on sexual media, masturbation and demisexuality:

> Due to me being demisexual, I personally do experience a frequent impact on my ability to masturbate. When using pornography as an aid for masturbation, I often experience difficulty actually finding material to use for masturbation, the reason I believe, being my lack of sexual attraction (since I almost only develop such after a connection) to the people featured in pornographic movies.
>
> On the other hand, I've instead found that pornographic art, comics and writings featuring established characters from media (from books, movies, TV shows, etc.) has been more effective as an aid for masturbation. This in turn I theorise then is due to me having made a connection to such characters. After all, the connection necessary for sexual attraction for demisexual people doesn't necessarily have to be a romantic connection; at least, I personally don't think this would have to be so.

These words suggest a side to demisexuality that I hadn't thought of before: the idea of this necessary, deep bond or emotional connection is well known, but I hadn't realised it might extend beyond interpersonal relationships.

A number of the people I spoke to mentioned masturbation; some preferred it as an alternative to sex with partners for whom they might feel deep love but not sexual attraction, while others rejected it as just another sexual activity they had no interest in. Again, attitudes towards masturbation varied more between individuals than it did across sexuality categories such as ace or demi.

DC, who uses the word aegosexual to describe her experience (specifically with regards to having fictional crushes), said she'd only ever met one person with whom she was comfortable enough to be physically intimate: her boyfriend. While DC said her experiences of sex with this person specifically were generally positive, she also added, "Aegosexuality and kink align in some very interesting ways and as it turns out sometimes having an extra pair of hands available can make things easier." This suggests that being physically intimate with another person might resemble assisted masturbation, more than our conventional ideas of partnered sex.

Looking broadly at the responses of the people I spoke to, this ambivalence or indifference towards sex was probably the biggest "universal" difference I could glean between asexual and allosexual people. When asked what she liked about being asexual, LL said, "I'm not sure there is something to like," but went on to add:

> But I think I like the freedom that comes with being ace, in regard to relationships. I don't know what it's like to want to have sex with someone who is not your partner. I can meet someone and have a relationship that is purely based on chemistry, not on sexual tension. I'm fine with my partner having sex

with other people, because it doesn't really matter to me. I feel like I have a different perspective on relationships.

Also, it makes my own romantic relationship different. My boyfriend and I's couple is not based on sex. We watch movies together, we have many activities that are purely non-sexual and not driven by attraction. Somehow, me having no sexual interest in him has made our relationship based on entirely something else. It's difficult to put into words. It's not like it's "pure" or something, because I don't believe sex is bad. I believe it feels good when it's done properly, when it's based on trust and fun. But sex is also, for me (and thus for us), an activity among many others. It kind of "de-dramatises" sex. It puts it into perspective. Sex is not a pillar in our relationship. It's an activity that makes us sweat and is not really practical, and I often prefer to watch a movie because at least I don't have to get naked. But it's an activity that we choose to do sometimes because we feel like it, not because we have to, not because "couples have to have sex, and have sex often when they are a young couple". It gives a certain value to our sexual activities.

And it makes our romantic relationship free of that sex injunction. There're no such things as cheating, or performance pressure. We don't care if we don't have sex often. We don't have conflicts over sex.

LL's words were echoed over and over by others. JH, when asked when and how she first realised she was grey-asexual, said, "being in a pandemic I'm realising how many risks people are willing to run for sex and it just...doesn't cross my mind in the same way". HBJ says, "I don't crave or need it in my life. I'm not suffering without sex or feeling a need to go on the prowl to find someone to scratch an itch," and went on, "I like the cuddling and pillow talk after sex even better than the sex itself."

VC, who is arospec asexual, used metaphor to conceptualise her attitudes towards sex and romance:

> Think of my ideal partnership as a cake (very ace of me haha) and that my recipe for the cake is different from the traditional cake recipe. In my recipe, sex is an ingredient that is briefly mentioned as an optional ingredient, maybe a topping. I don't really care for it but may be curious to try adding it to my cake at some point. In my recipe, romance is also listed as an optional ingredient, except I don't know what it is. I don't know what it looks like, how it tastes, and I would not know how much to add into the cake. If it was added to my cake, I wouldn't really be able to tell that it was in there because I cannot identify it. With utter confusion I would probably ask other people eating the cake if they can taste this ingredient. This is how unimportant these two ingredients are to my cake whereas a typical cake recipe would list them as essential.
>
> Meanwhile, for my demiromantic bisexual friend, their recipe is a meat dish. Romance to them is cornstarch, it tastes terrible on its own, but it is necessary in the recipe for the meat dish.

When discussing her past history of sexual behaviour LH, who is grey-asexual, said:

> I used to have sex with most people who asked me because why not? It's a free country! Nothing to lose? Why would you reject sex? And looking back it's crazy how much of an ace thing that was actually: I thought it made no sense to refuse strangers in bars because I felt the same amount of sexual attraction for strangers in bars as I do for people I like and care about: zero.

LH's experience almost inverts the conventional narrative of asexuality: she had sex willingly and often, not out of any real desire to do so, but because it was expected of her, and wasn't much different to any other activity someone might invite you to engage in. LH goes on to articulate the way that the sexual imperative, the idea that to be in a relationship – to be *human* – means having sex, influenced her own ideas and expectations, *even while she was in a relationship with another a-spec person*:

> I actually entered my current relationship not knowing I was ace; but by then, I was aware it existed. I was right in the middle of my gradual awakening, and I literally told her when we started dating: "just so you know, I'm not...crazy about sex... I don't do it that often" and she answered in a relieved tone, "Oh that's good! Me neither!" Then for weeks we dated and didn't have sex, and I kept thinking "Man, when she said she wasn't into sex either she really meant it...so are we...never going to have sex at all?"
>
> I mean when you read my other answers you must really wonder why that would bug me. But I was still so normalised! I kept thinking "I did say I didn't have sex a lot, but I didn't expect us to *never* have sex."
>
> After some time I realised that if we never had sex it was because neither of us ever asked it of the other and if that was the case, that was because neither of us actually wanted to have sex and we were both very much on the ace spectrum. Big shock for me to realise that: I felt we needed to be having sex despite never personally wanting to: I was just obeying my internalised command of "have sex because you are in a relationship"!

LH felt pressure to have sex with her partner, not because of anything her partner seemed to want, but because of what society wanted for the two of them. Whatever their personal sexual history, on the whole the people I spoke to seemed to simply not consider sex to be a *biological need* in the way allos seem to. Whether they did so or not, a majority said or implied that they *could* go without it.

The social expectations around what a relationship is supposed to involve can put pressure on both a-spec and allo partners, making it more difficult to actually identify what is going on: NO, who has been married to her husband for several decades, said that when she found out she was grey-ace, "I realised I had been blaming my lack of libido on my husband." If both she and her husband had had access to the concept of grey-asexuality from the start, NO's indifference towards sex might not have been a point of conflict.

This pattern of indifference is interesting because it somewhat contradicts the conventional way that we – even within the community – are taught to define asexuality. The presence or absence of sexual *attraction* didn't seem to be the most pertinent feature of asexuality for VC, LH, LL or JH, though it was for others. Even if they defined asexuality in the abstract in terms of attraction, the salient feature that united them seemed to be this ambivalence, the ease with which they could go without something that so many other people seem to think of as essential.

Sex repulsion

Note: This section contains discussion of sexual harassment, assault and childhood sexual abuse.

After ambivalence, repulsion seemed to be the next most common attitude people had towards sex: a number of people described themselves as sex repulsed or sex averse. SS described sex aversion in the following way:

> Some of us are sex positive, meaning we're cool hearing about sex or being around it. Some of us are sex neutral, meaning we don't care either way. Some of us are sex repulsed or sex averse, meaning we actively choose not to hear about sex, don't have sex ourselves, won't talk about it, don't look at porn or other sex-related media, and so on. Sex-averse people deserve to have our boundaries respected and not be exposed to sexual conversations, exposed to porn or touched sexually against our will in an effort to "fix us". That is abusive behavior. Respect the limits of all asexual people.

Hille *et al.*, the researchers who conducted the asexual sex survey, lumped sex-averse people in with those who were sex ambivalent, into a group they called "disinterest/disgust". Disinterest/disgust characterised 43 per cent of ace respondents, versus 19 per cent of grey-ace and 10 per cent of demi respondents. Responses labelled this way were unified by a *lack of interest* in having sex, with reasons ranging from a simple lack of desire to an active dislike or revulsion.

Among the people I spoke to in depth, though, disinterest and disgust seemed to make up two totally different – though sometimes overlapping – categories. Plenty of the people I spoke to who could be considered "sex ambivalent" were in fact happy to have sex if their partner wanted to, or if, as LL put it, they "felt like it". This was not the case for the sex repulsed. (Though Hille *et al.* did include the caveat that "there is an important distinction between wanting to and being willing to engage in these behaviors for individuals on the ace spectrum".)

Sex repulsion can manifest in innumerable different ways, and be connected to any aspect of sex and sexuality, abstract or concrete. It can be connected to bodies and embodiment, bodily fluids or touch-related hypersensitivity. It can also – per Hille *et al.* – be intertwined with feelings of ambivalence. AB says:

> I do not see the appeal of sexual activities except stimulating your body for like a minute. And sure that's great, but I can feel good by doing other stuff so why would I choose this over anything else? Watching other people have sex doesn't necessarily gross me out (sure having sex isn't the most beautiful scene anyway but that's not the issue) but it's rather that I realise that what drives these people to have sexual intercourse is something I will never be able to relate to. I simply don't get it. It's boring. I cannot feel the "passion" and "desire" that everyone talks about. Sex is nothing but a mechanical action because for me there is nothing else to it than performance: you're doing one thing in order to make your partner feel good and they return the favour. The connection that allos have to sex is something I do not understand.
>
> And that's why I would say my experience is rather "negative" [when asked if her experience of sex is negative, positive or mixed] because it doesn't bring me value: it's more of a hassle then a pleasure. Sex seems like a lot of work, no thank you!

The way AB describes her sex repulsion exemplifies the way many aces seem unable to relate to the passion or "spark" that many allos describe when talking about sex. The ways a person's sex aversion might manifest could vary a lot from person to person. SS described a fairly universal aversion:

> I don't discuss my sexuality right away with new people unless they cross a boundary, such as flirting with me or bringing up something they enjoy sexually in a way that infers that they

> would like to do that with me. If my boundaries are crossed, I will let them know that I'm grey-asexual and while I support their sexual activities, I don't want to hear about their sex life unless they are asking for my advice. The only people who have my permission to engage with me on a sexual level are my partners (right now I only have one monogamous partner). I am not comfortable having other people's sexual interest directed at me.

But others might experience aversion that was only intermittent, context dependent or linked to certain aspects but not others. OP, who describes herself as sex repulsed, says:

> Talking about the act of sex still makes me very, very uncomfortable. I once had a friend who was giving me pointers for a one-night stand, and she went into so much detail I just didn't know how to tell her how to stop. I was standing there like a deer in headlights just waiting for her to let me go. I do now understand that strategically placed cushions can help in getting everything into position for ease of access, which was nice of her and not something I ever thought about! Or want to think about!

CD, who is ace and demiromantic, says:

> I can recognize when my body has been stimulated in the course of my exercises (dilation treatments for vaginismus), but I dislike everything about it – I dislike the changes my body undergoes, and when I experience orgasm I find it unsettling. I am thoroughly repelled by the genitalia of both sexes and am awed and perturbed by the fact that people can be undone (and lives made and ruined) by something as basic as friction against certain body parts.

JH said, "There is literally nothing I would rather hear less than the sounds of people having sex in a nearby room." While EF's feelings of disgust or distaste, on the other hand, were specifically centred around bodily fluids: "I hate bodily fluids in any capacity. I think they're really gross. But I get that it's the connection between the individuals who are partaking that make it special for some people. I could go without having sex for the rest of my life."

EF's words echo AB's: sex, without the "spark", is reduced to wet body movements, and loses its "magic".

There were a number of people who expressed discomfort or aversion to various positions or ways of participating in sex. BC, who is demisexual, said:

> Giving in sex is really good. I really enjoyed learning my partner and reading his body and making him orgasm. But when it comes to my turn, I just shut down – I'm incapable of communicating and apparently look like I'm in pain. It feels painful sometimes, just way too much stimulation.

BC's words contrast sharply with LH's (grey-ace), who expressed almost the opposite attitude (though LH doesn't refer to herself as sex averse):

> I find penetration pleasurable, and it's one of the only reasons I went to male partners for sex back when I was sexually active. But the pressure to perform, to give the other person an orgasm, will always ruin it for me, haha. Basically, as I said, it's more of a chore than anything.

When asked what a partner can do to make her feel safe and supported during sex, she added:

> Leading the encounter. My lack of sexual attraction means that I feel very, very awkward during sex, because I'm just not that into it. Even if I'm finding the sensations pleasurable, if I'm expected to display my arousal to the other person, it feels horribly stilted and forced. I'm most comfortable in situations where the other partner plays a dominant sexual role (after establishing consent, obviously...) and is making the decisions, because this way I'm sure they're having fun and I can focus on what I want to get from the encounter.

It's important to note at this point that sex repulsion or aversion can change, developing or receding over time or in different circumstances. SS mentioned that it was important for her sexual partners to be:

> checking in regarding my boundaries and where I'm at in that moment in time. I might be interested in sex at 7pm, but sex repulsed by 9. Sometimes the window is very short. Sometimes I'm sex neutral or sex repulsed for months or years. Be respectful of that, recognising the fluctuation and accepting it without judgement or grumbling.

It's also important to remember that sex repulsion and asexuality aren't the same thing: HBJ, for example, says that nowadays, "I'm not riddled with trust issues. I'm not afraid of sex any more, haven't been for decades now...and I'm still ace."

One notable aspect of sex repulsion that I hadn't encountered before beginning this project was the idea of aversion specifically to being *perceived* as sexual, or being perceived as sexual in a different way from reality. Many people expressed discomfort at the idea of others seeing them as sexual beings, or with being an object of sexual desire. OP says of a previous relationship,

"Sex was tolerable, but I just thought it was a drag and I was so uncomfortable whenever he'd mention how sexy I was...," while DC said:

> I don't enjoy the experience of people perceiving me in a sexual way or involving me in a situation in which I am assumed to be allo. It gives me extremely visceral Nope vibes. From what I've heard from people describing gender dysphoria, it seems like a similar mechanism in terms of my interior identity and the outside world's perception of my identity being fundamentally mismatched.

I remember this idea cropping up in a casual conversation with a demisexual friend about fashion and clothing choice. My friend, who is very active within the wider LGBTQ+ community and dresses the part, recalled times when someone might make assumptions about them and their sexual preferences based on the clothing they wore, for example, assuming they were into BDSM or preferred a certain sexual role because they were wearing leather or chains. This made them very uncomfortable.

This discomfort with being perceived as sexual reminds me, as a trans person, of gender dysphoria. I can still recall being a younger, thinner-skinned babytran, and the visceral discomfort or even disgust that I used to feel when someone would make an assumption about my gender (and treat me accordingly) that was different from how I thought of myself and wanted to be perceived. Viewed in this light, this kind of sex aversion feels like a very reasonable reaction to being sexualised without consent.

The final pertinent dimension of sex repulsion that emerged from among my interviewees is a somewhat sensitive one: the idea of sex repulsion as a result of trauma. It's sensitive not only because of its connection to trauma, but because the idea of the "traumatised asexual" is one of the most widespread and enduring misconceptions around asexuality: the idea that all asexuals hate sex, and that something "happened to them" to make them this way.[5]

But out of the almost 40 people I spoke to in depth, only three or four mentioned specific trauma or abuse they had experienced within a context of sex and relationships linked to being sex repulsed – most of the sex-repulsed people I spoke to in fact took care to assert that they had no traumatic history that "explained it all".

And even for those who said they *had* experienced sexual trauma or abuse, and who had trauma responses that manifested as sex repulsion or touch aversion, there was no evidence that it had been the *cause* of their asexuality – though there is some evidence that, conversely, an asexual person might be statistically more likely to experience an unwanted sexual encounter, or more likely to interpret a sexual encounter *as* unwanted.[6]

SS, a sex-positive but occasionally sex-averse demi ace, said, "I have been the victim of violence and abuse because of my sexuality, specifically because I refused to have sex with men who became violent when rejected," but she did not explicitly name that abuse as a cause of her sex repulsion. This specific type of violence, which amounts to a denial of asexuality and sexual coercion, does not always "look like" what is conventionally considered assault, either. EF discussed a sexual relationship they had been in from the age of 15. When asked what they wished they'd known before entering into the relationship, they said:

> Where to start. This 22-year-old grown man should not be attracted to you. He should not be waiting for you to reach the AOC for the two of you to have sex – this puts pressure on you. You want to please him because he's waited so long even though

> you've said you're not sure how you feel about sex. And then, when you have sex for the first time and still have no interest and voiced that to him, don't let him persuade you that your feelings are just nervousness. This will make you second guess every interaction that you have for the next three years.

Even if EF's experience didn't involve physical assault, their former partner's predatory attitude that put pressure on EF to perform sexually when they didn't want to constitutes a pernicious kind of violence that had long-lasting ramifications.

CD experiences "post-traumatic stress disorder as the result of sexual abuse I suffered when I was young," which she specifically linked to a serious aversion to touch that lasted for many years. She goes on to say:

> For more than a decade, the illness sort of covered my asexuality, if that makes sense – I assumed that my lack of feeling had resulted from my experiences. But with time, and improved mental health, I was able to separate the two, to consider the "data points" indicating that I'd been disinterested in sexual matters even before my bad experiences.

DE, who had previously been married to an abusive partner, said, when asked about her experience of dating and past relationships: "Maybe if I had married a better person, it would have been okay. Maybe I would have been able to put up with the sex and maybe we would have been able to come to some compromise."

DE's experience of sex was inextricably tied to the unsafe space that she had been in when she had sex. In these cases – perhaps in most cases – an a-spec person's experience of and attitudes towards sex are dependent on context, life circumstances and how the people close to them, especially sexual partners, behave.

It's important to reiterate at this point that, while trauma responses *can* manifest as sex repulsion or aversion, I found no evidence of it causing asexuality: as I mentioned earlier, the majority of people who described themselves as sex repulsed did not mention any traumas that might account for it, and for those who did mention traumatic experiences, the connection was far more complex than cause and effect. HBJ, when asked at what point in a new relationship her a-spec identity comes up, said: "I still don't know if it was my orientation or my trauma that came up first, but I tended to be clear and up front about not wanting to be physically intimate with people. Massage yes, hand holding sure, cuddling great; kissing maybe; sex eek."

It may be impossible to fully detangle, for any given person, the true relationship between (a)sexuality and a history of trauma, and the assumption that trauma *causes* asexuality or sex repulsion is dangerous. It denies the idea of asexuality as a natural state and opens the door to a person's asexuality being pathologised. Aside from facilitating the othering and alienation of asexual people – and contributing to the idea of them as helpless, childlike or without agency of their own – it also potentially exposes them to harmful or invasive medical treatments.

It also occludes the very real existence – like CD, SS and HBJ – of asexual people who *had* experienced trauma and whose sex repulsion was connected, in *some* way, to that trauma. Survivors of sexual violence are among the most vulnerable in any demographic, and the community cannot be truly said to be safe unless a-spec survivors' voices are heard, even centred, in discussions of community issues.

But if research is done on the ace community by allos who assume that *all* of us are traumatised, it becomes impossible to study the actual relationship between sexual trauma, sex aversion and asexuality, an area of study that has received relatively little attention.

Sex-repulsed people simply *are*, and the connection between trauma, sex aversion and asexuality is complex and varies from person to person. Just as no one needs a reason to be gay, trans, straight or cisgender, no one needs a reason to be sex repulsed. And just as asexuality is not a disease to be cured, sex-aversion isn't a pathology unless the person experiencing it decides that it is.

Sex positive

Despite the prominence of sex-repulsed or ambivalent people among those I spoke to, there were just as many who said that they actively enjoyed sex, in one form or another – though unlike Hille *et al.*, I didn't ask anyone to define what they meant by "sex" before they spoke about it.

BH, who is asexual and on the aromantic spectrum, said, "I don't regret my sexual experience at all. For me, having sex helps create intimacy and deepens a relationship. Plus, it's enjoyable."

JTS, who is gay greysexual, says of his first sexual experience, "I felt loved and respected by the person I had sex with, so it was a memorable experience," and BH, who describes her previous experience with sex as positive, says that "talking beforehand about exactly what I'm comfortable with and respecting those boundaries, letting me set the pace, looking for enthusiastic consent throughout", were essential in making her feel safe and supported.

Hille *et al.* explored their participants' reasons for wanting or not wanting to have sex. They identified "emotional connection", "partner's desire" and "consent" as pertinent themes. Thirty per cent of asexuals, 40 per cent of grey-aces, and 70 per cent of demisexuals indicated that they needed an emotional connection – feelings of trust, intimacy and closeness – with a partner before they would have sex with them. Around 12 per cent of these answers also mentioned the importance of consent, negotiating boundaries or not wanting to feel pressured. Around 30 per cent of ace and grey-ace people, and 23 per cent of demi people, indicated that their desire to have sex was contingent on their partner's, with lots of overlap between the categories of emotional connection and partner interest.

These findings are pretty consistent with what my own interviewees said. For those who said they enjoyed having sex, three qualities emerged that they sought out in or required of their sexual partners: trust, respect for boundaries and communication. These three practices or qualities overlapped and intertwined considerably. For any one person it was often impossible to separate them, though all three might play a prominent role in that person's concept of relationships and intimacy: communication around boundaries; trust resulting from reliable, honest communication; negotiation of boundaries contingent on mutual trust between partners.

When asked whether her a-spec identity made it harder or easier to be in an intimate relationship, JH said, "I'd say harder. I am someone who has a hard time asserting herself and drawing boundaries, and my a-spec identity feels like just one more interpersonal roadmap I have to redraw." When asked whether she'd had a conversation with a past partner about her identity, she emphasised the importance of communication: "I didn't, and honestly I think if that had been part of the conversation the relationship would have had more of a chance."

BH said: "I've been in two sexual relationships, both before coming to terms with my a-spec identity. Luckily, I had two wonderful partners with whom I shared a lot of trust, so it was a very positive experience."

While HBJ, discussing her past experiences of sexual relationships, said:

> After being in a long-term relationship with the man who became my husband, I reached a point where I enjoyed sex as an extension of the intimacy we already shared as partners. I did feel comfortable enough and safe enough that I would initiate sex rather than waiting for my partner to approach me.

HBJ goes on to discuss the importance of a partner's respect for her personal boundaries – in this case, her freedom from pressure to have sex: "I guess I keep coming back to giving me time and space; I've said before, 'the freedom to say no is more likely to make me say yes', and that still holds true." Her words give the lie to the stereotype of asexuality as an inherently repressed or repressive identity: freedom from the pressure of compulsory sexuality is itself a form of sexual freedom.

There is no one single way for an ace person – even a sex-repulsed ace – to feel about sex. But the a-spec community, insofar as we are unwilling to compromise and are actively negotiating the shape of our relationships, is doing important work in figuring out how to navigate sex safely, not only in physical terms but also emotionally.

As I read through the anecdotes a-spec people had shared with me, I could imagine these conversations: *This is what I'm willing to do to satisfy your needs – any further and my autonomy is compromised. This is what I want us to explore together, and this is what I am happy for you to seek outside of our relationship. I know what we need to do to keep me safe, happy and comfortable, and your safety, comfort and happiness is equally important. Together, we find the lines we will not cross.*

Some of what I've said here may sound reminiscent of the language used in kink or BDSM circles. This is no coincidence: ace-spectrum people have been active in these communities for as long as they have existed,[7] and despite the vanilla assumption that it's just a kind of sex you wouldn't want your grandmother to hear about, kink and BDSM are less about finding interesting ways to orgasm and more about power, pleasure and heightening intimacy between partners – all within a safe, mutually negotiated environment.

To practise kink, it's necessary to build trust with your partner(s), communicate actively about what you want and don't want, and consistently respect your partner(s)' boundaries. So it's not surprising, perhaps, that there is considerable overlap between the two communities.

LG explained their relationship to kink as a grey-aroace person:

> I think to allos or people who don't have a basic kink education, the idea of aces being kinky might seem a paradox. But not all kink is sexual and even when it is, in BDSM there is context and a culture that respects boundaries and values consent so if aces want to explore things (or if they're just plain ol' kinky to be honest) they can do that in a place that feels safe. Or it might be that someone may not experience attraction or sexual desire unless there's kink involved. This applies for both aces and allos.
>
> I don't experience sexual attraction, but I do experience pleasure in my brain in other ways and sometimes seeing someone all dressed up in harnesses or latex can activate my brain in the same way. I may not be sexually attracted to them

> but seeing them like that makes my brain happy the same way it would be happy if I saw someone I thought was pretty.

When asked what a sexual partner does or can do during sex to make her feel safe and supported, SS said:

> Safewords! I love having a safeword. If at any point during sexual activity my libido fades or I start feeling sex repulsed or I'm just bored and I want it to be over, I can use our safeword to immediately stop everything that's happening and transition into aftercare where my partner will listen to me and accept feedback. This is a core part of BDSM that has helped me so much as an ace person, and the reason why I feel more comfortable dating or having sex with people educated in BDSM practices, especially SSC (Safe Sane Consensual) and RACK (Risk Aware Consensual Kink) philosophies.

The overlap between a-spec and kink community language is a fruitful one, offering potential space for members of both communities to build sexual safety and consent practices outside the "social scripts" of conventional relationships. And as it turns out, those qualities of mutual trust, respect for boundaries and communication don't just apply to sex: the closer I looked at the responses to other questions, on everything from allyship to alternative forms of intimate relationships, the more I could see those three qualities manifesting in different, often subtle ways. As I go on, I'll return to them periodically as a way of looking at a-spec identity not as a lack or negative quality but as a positive, mindful way of being.

Advice

I asked my interviewees if there was anything they wished they'd known before they had their first sexual encounter:

> Sex is a thing that you do not ever have to try if you don't want to. Your sexuality is what you say it is regardless of who you have or have not had intercourse with. HD

> Oh man, a lot of things I have in common with allo people, I think. That "you always bleed because you break your hymen the first time" is a lie, for one! And that you shouldn't try to have sex if your vagina's dry and tight from lack of arousal (sorry for how graphic that sounds). That lube exists and is okay to use. None of these things are specific to asexuals, but it's definitely worse when you're in the middle of convincing yourself you want it. But I guess I wish I'd known very early that sex is not a performance and I shouldn't try to act and look like I'm into it when I'm not. LH

> Complete darkness is *not* helpful, actually. EP

> The only thing that comes to mind here is a reminder that I was never broken, and that asexuality really is a thing all on its own. It might have been good to have real talk with other women about what sex could be like, but I was so fearful beforehand that I don't know if that would have helped, or just put me off the idea of sex forever! They say if you can't talk about it, you shouldn't do it, and I was super uncomfortable for a very long time even talking about it with anyone. I might have benefitted from listening while others discussed sex in an honest way, but I'm not sure. HBJ

That it's not that great? I mean, maybe it's because I don't feel sexual attraction. But sometimes, it's just a mess, I'm all sweaty, it feels good for five minutes and then I have to take a shower and go pee and it's like...was it worth the trouble? Also: longer does not mean better. LL

It's not all that much fun and it doesn't feel as good as advertised. Like frozen yogurt or hot yoga... I grew up believing the lie that sex would lead to happiness and the lack thereof caused sadness and depression. So as much as I really did not want to engage in the activity, I haphazardly pursued it until I discovered that having a best friend to share my life with was far more rewarding than the occasional orgasm and its less than satisfying denouement. NT

Having sex because you feel like it's the only way to keep a person is a bad idea and will make you feel worse. RR

Never had sex, but once I learnt that the majority of women don't orgasm from penetrative sex, I lost whatever little interest I had left. I'll stick to my very hardworking vibrator. RK

There are so many different types of condoms. If you're a person who's going to have a condom go into your body, you really should buy a bunch and start experimenting by yourself to see which ones feel okay for you. SS

That without "warming up" it can be painful and uncomfortable. Don't rush having sex or force someone to have sex. It's very different for everyone and the way society talks about sex as if it's a must in a relationship simply isn't true. These ideologies aren't healthy, especially if you aren't interested in sex in the first place.

The expectation and demand are there and it's harmful. It can make it more difficult if you're struggling to voice your identity or needs. Boundaries and acceptance are very important. HI

Don't feel pressured. Trust your gut. EF

Discussion questions

1. How do you *personally* feel about sex? Try if you can to completely strip away any of your attitudes towards sex that don't come from you organically. What I mean by this is, if there was no pressure at all from society, from friends, family, media, to engage in sex in one particular way, what would your sex life look like? Would it be different from what it is now? How different and in what ways?
2. Think about your own needs when it comes to sex. What is necessary in a sexual encounter, or more generally in a sexual relationship, for you to feel safe and comfortable? Was there anything described in this chapter that resonated with you?
3. Think about those three qualities of trust, boundaries and communication as they apply to your own sexual (or non-sexual!) relationship(s). Are all these things present in the way you'd like them to be?

The Future of Relationships

I've been seeing my current partner for about six months. We're both a-spec – and both busy – so we're taking it slowly. In the chapter on intimacy and romance ("What Is Love?"), I wrote about how I've been thinking more deeply lately about what intimacy and closeness mean to me. I've had the opportunity, while writing this book – and while dating a new person – to really think for the first time about what I want, what I want the future to look like and how to put that into words when I need to.

As a result, my partner and I have had a couple fraught – not in a negative way, but heavy – conversations where I've laid out some of the "stuff" I'd never said aloud to anyone before. I've been challenging myself to communicate: at the risk of sounding like a cliche, I'm trying to be radically honest. I've come to the conclusion that it's no good censoring myself, trying to hide my stuff or keep my needs a secret, because I'll have to make them known eventually. So I've been open about my boundaries and needs, including allowing myself to step away, to seek out solitude, to cancel plans when I've been tired or didn't have the energy for social interaction.

I'm still finding the whole process exhausting – and intimidating. No one teaches you how to do this stuff: you're just supposed to know how to get your needs across to the other person, or maybe you're supposed to hope your partner intuits them without you needing to put in the effort of communicating at all. But I left too much unsaid, I allowed my needs to go unmet too often, in my previous relationships – and let my partners do the same – so I am determined to put in the work.

And every time I've taken that leap of faith, each time I've (cringing inwardly) laid out some new need or worry, my partner has caught me, meeting me with understanding and compassion. I feel a sense of trust for my partner that has made our still-nascent relationship as rewarding as it has been challenging.

There are social scripts around dating and relationships, signals that a person is supposed to be able to send and understand. You're supposed to know what an "x" means at the end of a text message, and when to send one. You're not supposed to reply right away. You're not supposed to stay friends with your exes. I, like most a-specs and probably many queers, have never been good at understanding these norms. A straight, allo friend will text me about their relationship woes, the need to keep a new relationship secret from an ex or from co-workers, for example, or the obsession with which they're checking their partner's social media, and I'll be baffled.

When you're a-spec, and queer, it seems like all bets are off. You can U-haul after a month of dating, or you might see each other for a year and still not sleep over. I often feel like I'm feeling my way around in the dark – or like I'm blindfolded when everyone else isn't.

So I've had to train myself to put things into words, to ask questions, to make propositions, to ask my partner how they feel about something. Being a-spec and nonbinary has been good training: every step of the way I've felt like I've been putting into words things that other people have the luxury of never questioning. But I still often feel like there's no manual for my relationship. We're building it up from scratch, working out what to call each other, all the little gestures that remind the other person we're thinking of them. How to express affection and meet the other person's needs without relinquishing our boundaries.

At the end of the last chapter, I identified three principles or practices that seemed to characterise the relationships of the people I spoke to. The upshot of that chapter wasn't to say that ace-spectrum people need trust, communication or respect for boundaries *more* than allo people, but rather to say that the way we relate to sex and intimacy mean the stakes are higher for us. There is more pressure for us to insist on these things where we might otherwise have compromised. It means that relationships lacking these qualities can be all the more damaging, and that relationships that do have them can be sites of profound nourishment and healing – I myself am testament to this.

The more I've worked on the rest of this book, the more I've come to understand that sex and sexual health were only one context in which trust, communication and respect for boundaries was important to us, merely the context in which they were most apparent. In fact, these three qualities apply to most aspects of our interpersonal relationships, and indeed our interactions with the wider world.

So in this chapter, I want to pivot away from sex and explore a few types of intimate relationships that are not always sexual, not always romantic, but that *are* always conceptualised in a way that *queers* conventional ideas around sexuality, intimacy and coupledom. These types of relationships have already been adopted, adapted and explored within the a-spec community for years, and the people I spoke to discussed them as both real and ideal. Within these queer ways of being together intimately, the principles of communication, trust and respect for boundaries are put into practice in a constellation of overlapping ways.

Queerplatonic relationships

In 2010, an a-spec person called Kaz put up a post titled "A/romanticism" on their Dreamwidth page,[1] in which they lamented the difficulty of articulating their romantic orientation and what their ideal relationship would look like. Eventually they concluded that "What is your romantic orientation?" was in fact the wrong question to ask. Instead, they said that while they didn't want many of the trappings of romance, they still desired intimacy with someone they considered their BFF, just not in the way that is commonly expected from either close friends or romantic partners. They said, "my dream plan for my life involved living together with my BFF...possibly raising kids with her...and possibly marrying her for tax and visa reasons". Further, Kaz said they'd met a lot of ace or ace-spectrum people who "want a BFF who's also their life partner, they might want to live together with this person, they might want to raise kids together".

In the comments on this post, a number of terms were suggested, one of them being "queerplatonic" (by user Meloukhia), which other users quickly began to echo and adopt. In 2012 user Meloukhia, under the name SE Smith, wrote a longer description of queerplatonic relationships and what they meant to them and their QPP (queerplatonic partner):[2]

> I have several queerplatonic partners in my life, people with whom I'm deeply emotionally connected and in constant contact with...

> We share an intense connection that is complicated and rich and fascinating; we are, as a friend puts it, "in each others' pockets" and what's going on in their lives is intimately familiar to me.

Smith went on to say, of their local queerplatonic partner, "we function like a couple, we do things together, we are intimate with each other, though not necessarily in the way people expect. We are a couple."

A QPR is a relationship that "bends the rules" we use to distinguish romantic relationships from non-romantic ones. It typically involves more intimacy and closeness (physical or emotional) than what is considered normal or socially acceptable for friends. At the same time, it doesn't fit conventional ideas about what romantic relationships should "look like".

Despite the fact that the term was officially coined over ten years ago, I had never encountered it until I started writing this book and getting more involved with the a-spec community. A number of people used this word to describe relationships they were or had been in, or wanted, and many others described the sentiment without necessarily using the word itself.

VC says, "an alternative relationship I currently opt for instead of romantic relationships is a queerplatonic relationship. I would like to have a life partner". AQ says, "I'd love to have a partner and queerplatonic relationships at some point." And CF, when asked if there was anything she'd like to change about a-spec representation in the media, says, "It would be great to see in popular media a-spec characters with meaningful relationships be it strong friendships, queerplatonic relationships or romantic relationships to show that a-spec people are very well able to love and feel strong emotions."

Like "quoiromantic" and "alterous", queerplatonic is a term that attempts to describe the indescribable – indescribable because our received language doesn't accommodate it. AB, who is aroace, describes her first intimate relationship, which at the time she and her partner interpreted as romantic:

> For my first relationship, I wish we would have stayed in that "in between" phase where maybe for him we would have been romantic partners but for me we would have been something similar to queerplatonic partners (in a way, we were just close friends who enjoy spending time together, cuddling and occasionally kissing each other) and I'm sure it would have been perfectly fine for both of us. But instead, we needed to label it purely romantic and thus I had to conform to the expectations that came with it, which in the end ruined the relationship we had.

Had she and the people around her had access to the term queerplatonic at the time, AB and her then partner might have been able to stay together. Without the expectations others placed on them, they might have been free to explore a model of relationship that worked for both of them.

When asked, "What's something you'd like all allo people to know about dating someone with your specific a-spec identity?" AB said, "Nothing really specific, it depends for everyone and the type of relationship you would like to have ('fully' romantic or QPP, etc.). What's important is to discuss it with the potential partner and to set limits and boundaries that all parties respect." When describing her ideal relationship, she said:

> If I had a relationship (more like a queerplatonic relationship) with an allo partner who knows I'm a-spec and is 100 per cent okay with it; who would respect all my boundaries (and not use them against me); and who wouldn't expect something from me

> that I couldn't give them in the first place, then sure my identity wouldn't be any issue. (But it's rarely that simple.)

EF echoed these sentiments, saying, "If I was to date, it would be more of a queerplatonic partnership situation, which would probably be with another a-spec individual," and went on to assert that, "a QPR is not just having a best friend". When asked how the prospect of dating or entering a new relationship made them feel, EF said:

> I feel like having a QPR with another a-spec person would be lovely because all of the anxieties I would have about being in a sexual/romantic relationship probably wouldn't be there! There would be no pressure to do anything that I didn't want to do, and that would be really comforting.

Learning the word "queerplatonic" meant that some people, like AB, were able to look back and reinterpret relationships they had been in, and attraction they had felt, in the past. GH says, "for the longest time, I thought I was straight. Everyone I had ever been romantically in love with was a guy. Except for one person, I was never in any romantic relationship however, and even with that one guy, I now label it as queerplatonic." When asked if she'd ever been in a romantic and/or sexual relationship before, she said:

> More queerplatonic, really. It was stronger than friendship, but there was no romance or sex. I'm labelling it queerplatonic after the fact, but at the time, I thought it was romantic because I was in love with him, and he acted like he felt the same way, but never owned up to the label of boyfriend.

GH describes almost the opposite situation from AB: because the nature of the relationship wasn't something they communicated about at the time, and because what they had didn't fit conventional descriptions of romantic-sexual relationships, GH's then would-be partner didn't consider himself a romantic partner.

When asked if she'd like to be in a QPR again, GH said "Well, I'd like to be in a relationship that was clear from the start. I'd totally love another QPR, as long as both of us know it is one. In fairness, I never knew this term until 2017. Thanks, Tumblr!" If GH and her partner had both had access to it, the word queerplatonic itself would have allowed her to communicate better about the shape the relationship might take, and would allow both GH and her partner to draw new boundaries that conventional expectations around romantic relationships obscure or disallow. In other words, both parties consensually naming a relationship as queerplatonic would have enabled them to avoid, as EF puts it, "doing anything they didn't want to do".

While many people I spoke to said that they actively sought out or negotiated queerplatonic relationships with their partners, a number also used queerplatonic as a way of describing how they saw the world. RH, who is demiromantic, describes the way she'd felt attraction before meeting her current partner:

> Before that [developing romantic attraction to her partner] I would have described my attraction as a very close queerplatonic, in between platonic and romantic. I have been attracted to other people in this in between way before but can't really say for sure that I was romantically attracted to any one of them. I don't really know how I know, sorry!

Queerplatonic works not only as a model of an ideal queer relationship for many people but also as a conscious response to the "relationship hierarchy" that places sexual-romantic relationships above all others, and that frames the interplay between friendships, family and romantic intimacy as a zero-sum game, in which one type of bond in a person's life (usually platonic) must always lose out to another (romantic-sexual).

In the original post beneath which the term was coined, Kaz makes a point to say, "I worry that by calling my relationship and desired relationship 'in between friendship and romance' (which again feels a bit like I'm boxing it in) I'm trying to get relationship points from the hierarchy": Kaz's relationship with their QPPs is not best described in terms of the hierarchy. Rather than conceptualised as "in between" friendship and romance, which implies linear progress from friendship towards romance, the existence of *queer*platonic relationships – the hint is in the name – causes us to question the validity of the hierarchy itself.

But despite the fact that terms like queerplatonic, alterous and quoiromantic were coined and developed within our community, a-spec people are not the only ones to have conceptualised, and then rejected, that same hierarchy that says some people in your life should be more important than others. As Smith says of their QPPs, "Almost all of them are also in romantic sexual relationships in addition to their queerplatonic relationships with me, as well as other types of relationships with people in their lives."

I recently heard one of my (as far as I know) allo friends describe their flatmate as their "platonic ride-or-die". From the way they spoke about this person, it was clear they were "with" them in a very real way – emotionally, domestically – despite not feeling what we would call romantic or sexual attraction for them. I remember thinking that, like my interviewees' descriptions of their QPPs, what my friend and their flatmate had together sounded like an intense, caring, wonderful relationship.

So allo people can, and do, build relationships that are queerplatonic, or if not in name, relationships that at least queer what we would consider the boundary between platonic and romantic. In 2021, articles were published in the *Guardian*, *Refinery29* and *New Statesman*, all extolling the virtues of what they called romantic, intimate or passionate friendships.[3]

These articles – interestingly all written by women or femmes of colour – lamented the poverty in the English language's vocabulary around the big, messy, intense and often blurry boundary between friendship, love and intimacy. In "I'm single, but I get all the romance I need from my friendships", Tšhegofatšo Ndabane says, "I expect my relationships to be founded on a deep and sacred friendship." Writing about getting into a committed relationship – and eventually breaking up – with her best friend, she says, "I wanted to 'do life' with her...the only thing that changed [when they got together] was that we began planning for a future together."

Ndabane goes on to discuss the ways that the relationship hierarchy, and the strict line heteronormative society teaches us to draw between romance and friendship, harms people of all orientations by – like AB and her first partner – creating strict expectations around this or that type of relationship and telling us the relationships we have are deficient if they don't live up to those expectations. Says Ndabane, "One reason we'd lose a friendship in a breakup is if our expectations of romantic partners are vastly different from the expectations we have for our friends."

In "Romantic partner? Who needs one when it's friends who truly help us get through life", Sonia Sodha discusses her disillusionment with normative expectations around "happily ever after". Among her diverse group of friends, Sodha says, "the thing we have in common is how much we rely on our friendships with each other to get through it all". Like many a-spec people I've spoken to, Sodha describes spending her twenties "searching for the love of my life", only to realise that:

> a happy romantic partnership that lasts a whole lifetime is probably something only a minority of people will ever achieve. Sustaining a lifetime relationship is actually quite an advanced emotional skill and, for various reasons, relating but not limited to their childhood and early adulthood experiences, it's one lots of people don't have.

Friendships, not romantic partnerships, are the enduring and nourishing relationships in Sodha's life. So, too, for many of the people I spoke to – and for myself.

In "What is romantic friendship", Hirji and Krishnamurthy write about both their own relationship – a passionate, enduring friendship – as well as the relationship between Iris Murdoch and Philippa Foot. The relationships they describe are in between, or entirely apart from, both romance and conventional friendship and only inadequately described by either of these words. But whereas Murdoch and Foot struggled to find language to describe what they had between them, Hirji and Krishnamurthy have the phrase "romantic friendship", and, perhaps more importantly, the insight that their relationship need not fit into one "box" or another in order to be real or long lasting: "Ultimately, deep, lasting love comes in many forms."

The word "queerplatonic" offers an opportunity to anyone who encounters it, an invitation to develop a more nuanced understanding of the relationship between platonic and romantic attraction, desire and relationships.

And unlike "romantic friendship", queerplatonic also asserts its queerness on its sleeve. It draws a direct connection to other subversive or non-normative ways of being a family, being intimate, being committed, and to a community that has formed around marginalised experiences of romance, sex, desire and attraction. Anyone may enter into a queerplatonic relationship, anyone may experience queerplatonic attraction, but the people who have pioneered this language, and who have been exploring these types of relationships, are part of that history. By using the word queerplatonic to describe these relationships, that history is also being honoured, and the already wide boundaries of the queer community expanded further.

Polyamory and relationship anarchy

In an article[4] for a-spec magazine *AZE Journal*, writer and researcher Jo Ross-Barrett describes their experience of being in a polyamorous, anarchic relationship with multiple partners: "the only way I can make sense of relationships is that they are what the people in them want them to be".

As an autistic, asexual person, Ross-Barrett realised early on that most of the conventions that guide how we enter into and behave within intimate relationships didn't work for them. It didn't make sense that their valued friendships should take a backseat to a romantic or sexual relationship, or that they could kiss or be physically affectionate with some people but not with others – and so they're a strong advocate for "taking each relationship on its own terms and on its own merits".

It also didn't make sense to them to be with only one partner. Unlike "queerplatonic", a newish term mainly used in a specific niche, the concept of polyamory is already in the popular consciousness. Indeed, it has almost the opposite problem: a surfeit of cultural baggage. Simply put, ethical polyamory[5] acknowledges the value of multiple relationships in a person's life, and assumes that love is not a finite source. It's based on mutual consent, communication and equality, actively negotiated between all parties in the relationship, whatever form those connections take.

But for most of us in the Anglophone West, the word probably calls to mind media depictions of hippie communes, suburban "swingers" gossiped about in hushed tones, bigamous Mormons or "secret second wives". It's a word associated with various transgressions of the romantic-sexual social order; it challenges the idea that each person has a single "soulmate", and that to be "faithful" to a partner means foreclosing the possibility of caring for anyone else.

At the same time, it seems like every third person on OkCupid has "ethical non-monogamy" in their profile, and more and more popular media is depicting happy, healthy, unconventionally coupled relationships.[6] It seems as though the norms around "fidelity", and the primacy of the nuclear family, might be shifting – though only in specific contexts.

One of these contexts is the a-spec community. Of the people I spoke to, when asked to describe their ideal relationships, a number mentioned polyamory as a way for their or their partners' needs, both physical or emotional, to be met without putting strain on the relationship. SKW, for example, said of his current, committed partnership, "Our relationship...is polyamorous in nature, and...we could date more people if we were to feel the need, or came to meet someone special."

Part of what makes polyamorous relationships so ideal for people on the ace spectrum is that they acknowledge the idea that no one person needs to fulfil every one of their partner's needs: for someone who isn't comfortable being available for their partner in all the ways a conventional romantic relationship would require – especially if fulfilling those needs would cross a boundary they're not comfortable crossing – the presence of a third partner, just as valued but emotionally or physically available in a different way, is ideal.

LH describes the way that a practice of polyamory would be essential to the long-term health of the relationship:

> We once opened the relationship, back when I moved six hours away from her for a year, so I hope that talk doesn't go too bad, but it's a bit stressful to think about. It's not strictly connected to our asexuality, it's just another part of my identity. I think for me, being able to experience crushes or date around or maybe even have sex if at some point in my life I want to (and I have at times wanted to) would make it more likely that I'll remain 100 per cent happy with and grateful for what I have with her.

LH doesn't experience jealousy in the conventional sense:

> I don't like the idea that possessiveness and jealousy is legitimate when in a relationship... I know I'm happy with my current asexual relationship, but I also know some people would not differentiate it from a partnership or friendship if I don't want to have sex with my partner nor want to forbid her from having sex with others... I don't know, it makes it weird for me.

While Ross-Barrett says they also haven't experienced jealousy, they can understand why some people might have an instinctual, visceral reaction to seeing a partner be intimate with someone else. And while this reaction may be overcome given time, this is where those tenets of communication and trust, so strongly advocated for no matter what type of relationship they were in, are so important.

While in a conventional monogamous relationship, trust might revolve mainly around remaining faithful to your one partner, in a polycule, with more moving parts, trust is a bit more complex and multilayered. It encompasses trusting your partner to communicate to you any needs of theirs that aren't being met, giving you both the opportunity to have a conversation about it – potentially looking for a new partner to add what is missing. But it also means trust around sexual health, practising safe sex and making sure you're not accidentally exposing your partner to an STI without their knowledge (as often happens when one half of a conventional couple is unfaithful). As Ross-Barrett says, "part of ethical polyamory is taking responsibility for protecting your partners' wellbeing in terms of sexual health".

But this sense of responsibility for your partners' wellbeing extends beyond sexual health, to a general sense of taking responsibility for your own actions within a relationship. With more than one partner, the stakes are higher and there are more chances for someone to get hurt if there isn't active communication and a solid foundation of trust.

This is where the concept of relationship "anarchy" comes into play: a philosophy of relationships built around examining – and, when necessary, setting aside – the social norms surrounding all aspects of intimate relationships. Coined in 2006 by Andie Nordgren,[7] relationship anarchy is a style of being intimate with others that is adjacent to polyamory, but doesn't necessarily assume multiple partners – indeed, a hallmark of relationship anarchy is that it doesn't necessarily assume *anything*. It takes the premise of communication, trust and mutual negotiation and bakes it in from the start, allowing everyone involved to build their relationship from the ground up.

Ross-Barrett recounts making up handouts for potential new partners, including definitions and FAQs about relationship anarchy. In a hypothetical conversation with this prospective significant other, they might say, "Hey, you seem really cool, and I like you a lot – I'm not sure exactly how I want to express that yet, but would you be interested in spending more time together?"

Rather than having any set expectations about what the other person might want – and rather than proceeding according to a "script", where miscommunication is a real possibility – they simply express their desire to get closer to the new person in *some way*: "instead of assuming what 'a relationship' is, you talk about it". Nothing is assumed a priori and so anything is possible.

If this doesn't sound very romantic, that's no coincidence: much of the basis of relationship anarchy is based around actively cutting through the thicket of social norms – the "scripts" surrounding how we're taught to go about courtship and romance – that dictate the ways we should be intimate with each other, from "rules" about fidelity to questions of who should bear children and participate in parenting. Ross-Barrett says, "it's all about asking and agreeing on things, rather than assuming them from a shared concept of a 'prototypical' relationship model".

Because they're both based on an idea of active negotiation between partners to ensure everyone's needs are met, polyamory and relationship anarchy are closely interlinked: many people who practise ethical non-monogamy consider themselves relationship anarchists, and vice versa. And both practices rely heavily on what my interviewees prized so highly when it came to their relationships: trust, communication and respect for boundaries.

Over and over while I was reading Nordgren's manifesto for relationship anarchy, I was struck by how familiar some of the things she was advocating for sounded. Indeed, "trust is better" is seventh on the list, and "change through communication" is number eight. "Love is not more 'real' when people compromise for each other because it's part of what's expected" reminded me of the people I'd spoken to who had worked so hard to, in spite of all the normalised expectations to "put out" or perform sexually for a partner, find partners who would respect their boundaries around sex or physical intimacy. Nordgren also advocates freeing ourselves "from norms dictating that certain types of commitments are a requirement for love to be real, or that some commitments like raising children or moving in together have to be driven by certain kinds of feelings". If that doesn't describe the ideal a-spec relationship, I don't know what does.

Like queerplatonic partnerships, non-monogamous and anarchic relationships are already being practised – in some form or another – both inside our community and out. They're not new, either: people of all sexualities have long been finding relationships that work for them, often on the margins of society. We didn't invent them, only taken what is useful to us and discarded the rest.

Perhaps, with the shape of society changing and economic forces giving each of us an increasingly globalised, transient existence, relationship anarchy – or something like it – will become the norm. As many of us are, for the first time, given the chance to *choose* whether to pursue a conventional family or set it aside in favour of something else, relationships like Jo Ross-Barrett's will become so commonplace they no longer need to be named. Perhaps everyone – ace, allo, gay, straight or bi – will be able to ask for, and get, what they need.

Discussion questions

1. Had you heard of queerplatonic relationships before reading this book? In what contexts? What about relationship anarchy?

2. How do you tell the difference between a friendship and a romantic relationship?
3. Thinking of "monogamy preference" like one of Chu's "components of intimacy", what is your monogamy preference? If you've never been in a non-monogamous relationship before, would you consider it? Why or why not?
4. If you're not comfortable with the idea, do you think you might be more comfortable if the conventions, norms and expectations around relationships were different? What would have to change in order for you to be comfortable?
5. If you were to consciously enter into an anarchic relationship (if you're not in one already!), what would that look like for you? Thinking more generally, if there was no societal pressure to be monogamous, or to prioritise romantic-sexual relationships over friendships, what do you think your most committed and intimate relationship(s) would look like? Who would it be with?
6. Nordgren advocates "find[ing] your core set of relationship values": How do you wish to be treated by others? What are your basic boundaries and expectations of all relationships? What kinds of people would you like to spend your life with, and how would you like your relationships to work? What are some of your core relationship values?

Joy

> I was in a supermarket and there was a gift box of (I think) Wine Gums sweets, each box had a different little message on it, one of them said "You're ace!" (meaning ace as in cool/great), so obviously I sent a pic to my friends saying "just got outed in Home Bargains". EH

I ended the previous part of this book with a look at the ways a-spec people have been building relationships for themselves from the ground up, finding ways to communicate about our needs and boundaries – and to make sure our intimate partners know what they are.

But when it comes down to it, for a lot of us living as a-spec means coming to understand that we are, on our own, enough. We don't need any one relationship, any one partner, to be complete, and the things that make us unique should be embraced and celebrated, not pushed aside under the pressure to do what everyone else is doing.

Solitude is important to me. If I spend too many days in a row at my day job, attending events or socialising, I begin to feel like I'm being pulled in too many directions at once, and without some time to be alone with my thoughts I feel like I start to forget who I am.

At times like these, even being around the people closest to me can be too much, and the only solution is to spend a day (or at least an afternoon) on my own, gathering myself up again. These habits are easier to maintain in spring and summer, when the green space around Edinburgh becomes lush and welcoming, or in autumn when the parks of Edinburgh are crowded with interesting fungus. In winter I make do with projects around the house that use my hands, allowing my thoughts to ramble free.

I've felt this need for solitude for a while, I think, in one form or another, but it's only very recently that I've been able to recognise it not as a problem but as a fundamental part of who I am, part of what makes me, me. Why did it take me so long? It took me this long because my whole life, I had never been told that solitude is something you should *want*.

I grew up thinking that, because of my identity – an identity I constantly hoped would simply go away on its own – I would be alone forever. I thought that even if I found someone, at a certain point, I'd fail to give them what they want and they'd leave. This gave me – and lots of people like me, I'm sure – something of a complex: even though I craved solitude and needed space to centre myself, I became terrified of doing anything on my own.

I spent half a year in Ireland in my third year at university. This was my first time living so far away from home, and I didn't know anyone in the city I was going to live in. I made friends quickly, some of whom I'm still in touch with, but when it came time to travel to the continent and see Europe (coming from California, I didn't know if I'd ever get another chance), I couldn't find anyone to go with me. I spent that week dragging my backpack through Prague, Vienna and Nice, chased by a sense of profound loneliness. I realised this loneliness was always with me to some extent; I was always trying to ignore it, but it only came out when I felt very alone. It wasn't just loneliness in the physical sense – away from home, friends, significant others: it was also a feeling of aloneness in *who I was*.

Years later, when I got into a relationship for the first time since coming out as a-spec, my fears were assuaged: I finally had someone to do things with, someone to plan a future with. And even if I did travel or do activities on my own, I wasn't *really* alone because I had a partner, so that was okay. Getting into a relationship validated me in a way I hadn't known I needed.

Then the pandemic came around, and the UK locked down. I started spending most of my time at my partner's place, my first time living with a significant other, without a space to call my own. Almost immediately, I started craving the solitude I'd once been so fearful of – and I felt guilty whenever I felt the almost visceral need to be alone. I'd be fine for a while, but at a certain point, without being able to explain why, I would have to flee, returning to my own flat and my own bedroom, my solitary walks in the woods.

Predictably, this need for solitude – and my inability to explain why I needed it – put a strain on our relationship. And when we eventually broke up, one of the ways I was able to care for myself was by finally embracing it, taking time for just myself in a way I never had before. I'm convinced now that, at the height of the pandemic, those long walks in the woods or bike rides to the beach were the only thing that kept me from going completely insane. Time alone in nature became an essential part of my routine when I was feeling stressed or distracted or anxious, which in 2020 and 2021 was pretty much every day. And along with lots of work done in therapy, I was able, maybe for the first time in my life, to start figuring out who I am *when I am on my own*.

I've heard from lots of people who, after breaking up with a long-time partner, find themselves on the rebound, desperate to find a new one. It's difficult to sit with oneself if, like me, you weren't used to doing it comfortably, and lots of people I've spoken to have found it hard to know who they are when they're not in a relationship. After all, we're taught that being in a (sexual, romantic) relationship is the most important and fulfilling thing a human being can do – and it's treated as perfectly acceptable for someone to base their entire personality around their status as part of a couple. Women, especially, are encouraged to subsume their identity to that of a male partner.

So what is a person supposed to do if being in a relationship, for whatever reason, isn't an option for them? How are we supposed to know who we are as self-contained beings, with our own needs and wants, totally separate from anyone else's, when everyone is telling us we're incomplete?

Part of the whole point of this book is trying to answer that question, but I still don't know. Even I wasn't able to start figuring it out until I'd done tons of work in therapy and, yes, started writing this book. The most important thing I've realised since doing all this work is that solitude isn't scary. It might mean something frightening, like the prospect of not having a loved one around or of moving to a new place, but it's not inherently a bad thing.

For many people, being alone symbolises a failure to live up to the aspirational life that society tells them they should want. It certainly did for me. But I'm no longer afraid of that: in fact I see it as more of a strength than a failure. If I end up uncoupled, then so be it. I'll still have close friends, my career, the beauty of nature to enjoy. And if I end up staying with partner, then I know I'll be able to embrace her wholeheartedly because I want to, and not because I'm afraid of being on my own.

There's nothing inherently bad about ending up on your own: we are all whole people all by ourselves. No matter what connections we find for ourselves – close friendships, a spouse, children or relatives – no other person completes us. We are each of us complete already.

When I say "a-spec joy", I'm talking about understanding – and believing – that regardless of what kind of relationship you are in, or what kind of feelings you feel, you are complete as you are. Believing that if you don't feel sexual attraction, don't form romantic bonds, it's not because you're missing something but because you are feeling something else. Some other kind of passion, some other desire or need, that still exists even if we don't have a word for it yet.

I'm writing this chapter just after my final session with a therapist I've been seeing for almost a year. Today is a day of endings: this is the last chapter I'll be drafting in a book I've been working on for two years. But both of these endings also feel like beginnings, like I'm laying the groundwork for future projects, further growth. Instead of something that was happening to me and is now coming to a close, both reaching my final therapy session, and the prospect of putting down my pen and sending this manuscript to my editor, are the culmination of years of hard work.

And because this ending is a beginning, and I'm looking forward to sharing this book with the world, joining the conversation around the a-spec community as it moves into the future, I wanted to make a choice to end this book on a positive note.

In an Ace Week article celebrating Black asexuals,[1] grey-a creative Grace B Freedom said:

> My grey demi asexuality is not about what I am without but more like where I am full. My asexuality is embodied. My grey demi aceness is Black AF, is nonbinary AF and queer AF. My grey demisexuality is aesthetic, spiritual/emotional, and sensual attraction forward and exists inside of the immeasurable

> yearning to be present to unplumbed emotional connections. It shows up as interdependence and curiosity inside of intimate connections that are reciprocal, where I can practice the vulnerability of my wholeness. While the seat of my erotic does not rest on the legs of white supremacist cis heteropatriarchal allosexuality, there is indeed an erotic seat and it is indeed hot.

This quote resonated with me because it was the first time I had seen being a-spec described in such a consciously, radically positive way. Grace describes their grey demi asexuality as *embodied*, made up of new types of intimate connection – connections *not yet discovered* in mainstream romantic sexuality. Their a-spec identity is exciting new territory. This is what I want passionately for my community. I – like Grace – am tired of talking about what other people think we are missing: lack of attraction, refusal of certain kinds of relationships.

Instead, I want to explore the things that make me happy to be a-spec, proud to be a part of my community. A-spec joy is about embracing ourselves as we are and finding joy and pleasure in our own unique way of being in the world.

I asked the people I spoke to, "What do you like about being a-spec?"

> Being aroace, I did a lot of work in unlearning that my worth as a person was connected to finding a partner. I don't feel the need to prove my worth by having someone find me attractive or want to date me. Being single all my life is not a sign of loneliness or failure for me, it's just my natural state. I would love to be a single crazy cat lady, allergies permitting. LG

> I like that my partner and I get to build our relationship around what works for us, and what we want it to look like, it's easier

to avoid falling into the traps of this is what relationships are supposed to look like [by] default. I like that I get to form close, loving relationships with people that aren't my partner without having to worry about jealousy or overstepping arbitrary social rules. I like that my partner and I get to work out our own language for showing each other support and affection, without the easy fall back of sex and sexualised language. I like knowing that my partner is dating me because he likes dating me, not because I'm pretty and we have sex. KL

The realisation made me a lot less concerned about the future of my relationship with my partner after they came out as trans, since I realised my romantic feelings and sexuality were a lot more complex than just "straight" or something along those lines. It has made me a lot more open to the idea of sexless dating (especially since I also am polyamorous as well, this has been a welcome realization). Thereby affirming my already existing opinion that a singular partner shouldn't have to be able to cover all of their partner's needs, nor should they be expected to. SKW

I love being on my own, I love being the one person who determines my life and not being tied to anyone. LV

I like that I'm incredibly attracted (romantically) to personalities and that sex is something that is special and about being with the person. People who hook up are also extremely valid though! Slut-shaming is dead. RR

I like knowing that I'm not attracted to anyone, and that I don't want to have sex – I find it comforting to have that as something I currently know is true about myself and therefore don't need to worry about particularly. Instead of being stressed about if I should feel something, I can focus on being okay with the fact that I don't. IJ

It feels a little like a superpower to live without getting caught up in sexual desire all the time! BH

It's freeing, in a way. To not have to think about relationships, to not have to look for someone to fall in love with. To not be dating. It's just really nice. I can work on my personal projects without any worry. It's quiet. I can buy some plants, maybe think about adopting a cat... I can help my friends, I can laugh at myself when sexual innuendo goes over my head, I can ignore people flirting because I genuinely don't pick up on their signals. Saves a lot of stress! OP

I do feel that I'm able to make more rational decisions about difficult things such as choosing partners, when to introduce sex into a relationship and ending relationships. I am not as attached to sex as allosexual people, and I'm less distracted by it. I am more patient and sensitive than the average allosexual person. I have taken more time to educate myself, and I'm less judgemental. I'm more willing to help others explore their sexuality and find their labels and identities. I'm more open and supportive of other marginalised people. SS

...my romantic relationships don't have the pressure of "good sex" to work. My partners don't have to give me an orgasm for me to consider them valuable and compatible partners. It simply doesn't factor in. And one final, terribly down-to-earth thing: back when I was sexually active, there were so many fears and health concerns. People keep talking about how healthy it is to have a sex life, but I have not had any UTIs or yeast infections since I stopped being sexually active, to say nothing of pregnancy scares. Staying healthy is much easier without a sex life! LH

I like that it has widened my understanding of the variety of ways in which people can care for each other, and that all are of equal worth and validity. CD

I like the community. I like being close to other a-spec people and having this in common with them. I think diversity is amazing and I love learning ways in which other people differ from myself. I have a perspective on love and relationships that I feel helps me understand the world better and makes me more open to other people's differences. HD

The a-spec communities have done so much work around dismantling allo and amatonormativity, and we offer such a powerful lens through which to view the world. Not taking sexual and romantic attraction as a given and thinking about kinds/elements of attraction differently is incredibly impactful. EL

I like having a structure to understand and describe how I feel, and knowing that others have felt the same way. I like knowing I'm not just wrong or broken. RH

There is something freeing about saying "fuck it, I'll just be me" and not letting the pressure of society rule your life and dictate how you should be. I love the ideal of punk and voidpunk and my identity is radical and political in itself. As an aroace, your existence goes against some of the biggest social norms in Western society: hetero- and amatonormativity. I'm punk because I'm aroace and I love that. My pure existence challenges society

> and even though that also means I'm a threat in its eyes, I love being aroace. AB

When I talk about a-spec joy, I'm talking about the ways that we are empowering ourselves to change our own points of view. If we want to see our orientations not in terms of "less than" or lack, but instead as unique and valuable ways of being in the world – if we want to find the ways of being that fulfil our needs and desires – we must unlearn what we have been told about ourselves.

I'm a little suspicious of the word "identity". As a trans person, I'm used to it being used as something of a sop, with people referring to my "gender identity", while the cis people around me get to simply *be* a man or a woman. I don't want to be in a situation where we talk about an a-spec identity without also acknowledging that allosexuality and alloromanticism are also identities.

So while I've written this book I've continually questioned my own use of the word and what I mean by it, while admitting that in many cases there is no better way to refer to my subject matter. I need "identity" if I want to talk about community, about a positively constituted a-spec *culture*, from ace memes and cake jokes to the visual art and fiction that so many of the people I spoke to mentioned they were creating.

More and more, the visible face of the community is changing. A far cry from scandalous early 2000s talk-show interviews, and the implicitly-ace-but-really-just-repressed nerds of mid-2010s TV, today, we're starting to see a-spec people represented in media that we ourselves have created, or at least been consulted on. Works of art are being created that represent ace, aro, demi and grey-a people as passionate, caring, complete humans.

A-spec rep is still not perfect: even as we are making art, allo people are still telling our stories for us. Most stories featuring people uninterested in romance or sex still frame that as a bad thing. Friendships never last, or if they do they become romances. Characters who could be happily a-spec still settle down, grow out of it, find "the one". And most of the stories with explicit representation are still asexual-specific. Aces are still portrayed as mostly white, cis and alloromantic, or as aliens and robots – and even if we're not, we're still seen as humourless and socially inept, the butt rather than the teller of jokes. And at the end of the day, sex and romance are still central to most pop culture storylines – and literature, and advertising, and news – and this will probably be true for a very long time.

But the landscape is changing, in large part thanks to the tireless fight of a-spec activists, creatives and researchers who've been telling our stories and combing the archives for traces of our history. Slowly, we have been proving to the world that we have always existed. Like distant stars, we've not always been visible, but we were always there. We fought on the front lines of the early LGBT movement,[2] alongside others whose sexualities were "betwixt and between". Our history stretches backwards in time, through the non-normative couples of Boston marriages, through the Golden Orchid society,[3] the group of Qing Dynasty women who rejected marriage and heterosexual sex. We have been among those who chose solitary or monastic life since before recorded history, our self-concepts changing as mainstream ideas of sexuality and romance have changed.

Over the years, we have tried to find places to be without apology. I want this place, here, right now, to be one of them. It does feel like times are changing. We are teaching the world our language, we're making art for and about ourselves, that reflects the fullness, the vibrant creativity and diversity of our community. I am able to speak to and share my story with young people who are going through what I went through alone. Of course, history isn't a linear story of progress. Our political moment will change, and we may lose each other again. But for now, it feels like we're stepping into the light.

One of the best things about coming out, and about finally taking the plunge and openly owning my identity, is that it's allowed me to connect with people around me who I hadn't realised were on the same journey. Over and over, writing this book, I've been reminded how privileged I am to get to speak to so many people like me, to get my head above the murky waters of allonormativity, to bridge the gap of silence between myself and my quietly a-spec friends. I think again of the Halloween party, where we all stayed up until 2am because none of us wanted to leave – the joy of realising that, by sheer coincidence, most of the people in the room, friends we'd invited, were on the ace spectrum like me.

When I first realised I was ace – before I even had a word for it – I made an unspoken assumption that I would never meet someone else who understood. I assumed that whatever it was I was learning about myself would always be an invisible barrier between me and the people around me. So writing this book – learning our community's language, learning the little signs by which I have learned to tell when someone is "like me" – has made the impossible possible. It made it possible for me to find people who not only understood but who needed that connection as much as I did.

I spent years thinking that being a-spec would push people away from me, so it's hard to put into words just how important it is that my being a-spec, and talking about it openly, has deepened some of my closest friendships. I have heard the relief with which some of the people I've spoken to have embraced the language I've given them: it has been an immense privilege.

Being a-spec has allowed me to form connections where I had thought there would be only lack.

In the spirit of that connection, I thought it would be most fitting to give the a-spec people who shared their experiences with me the last word:

"What is some advice that you would give to your younger self, or to another person with your identity, who is just starting to figure things out?"

> Don't be someone you are not to please others. NT

> You are enough on your own. You don't have to base your self-worth on having a significant other. GH

> It's okay to be different. Sometimes it might be hard, sometimes you might feel like you're missing out on this wonderful thing that everyone else gets, but you aren't. Being ace is its own wonderful thing. LM

> Stop waiting for it to happen. It's not going to happen, so just go and have fun, and pursue your own interests. RK

> You are not alone. Find your people. You are not broken. LV

> Most straight people don't agonise over whether or not they are straight. Most allo people don't agonise over whether or not they are allo. If you are thinking or worrying about it significantly, it's worth exploring... You're best to look into a-spec communities themselves, rather than just what other people are saying about them. And when exploring your attraction in real life, if you feel

you can, it is absolutely best to communicate clearly with your partner or someone else you trust about how you are feeling. RH

Whatever things you wish could be part of your future, that can be what you work towards. You don't have to try to fit your life into the template you've been given, you can create your own. EL

Just because every form of media you consume says that romantic love is the pinnacle of human connection doesn't mean it is required to live a happy, fulfilling life. Friends are awesome. EP

...focus on what feels like it will help your life practically, and the people you interact with, rather than worrying about exact details or the need for neat definitions. Identity isn't just an abstract concept, it is real and rooted in material conditions, so think about what will make you feel happy and allow you to build the life you want, for example, does a particular label help you know and define who you want to be and be seen as.

Also, talk to people! Especially about the things you're worried about or unsure of. You don't need to have anything worked out to talk to someone else about it – you can say "I don't think I'm ever attracted to anybody", for example, and take it from there.

And allow yourself to imagine a future in which you are happy and comfortable with who you are. It's not something you're not allowed, and it'll help you work out what you want in life. IJ

Identifying as a-spec doesn't have to be a permanent thing, so don't feel pressure to wait until you're positive... It's okay to date and figure yourself out. BH

Life's all about learning about yourself, there's no shame in not being certain. RR

There's no gatekeepers to sexual orientation. If you identify as asexual, nobody has the right to tell you that's not who you are. LL

One, give yourself space. Two, don't listen to people who have never heard about asexuality about whether or not you are asexual. Three, just...be patient with yourself and don't be afraid to assert your boundaries no matter what. JK

Just be kind with yourself. Accept yourself and try not to fear other people for not being tolerant with what you are. JTS

You are not weird or broken, you are not waiting for the right person, you're not immature or a late bloomer. And you are not alone. Even though society sometimes tells you otherwise, other forms of love such as friendship or family are as important, as powerful, as deep as romantic/sexual relationships. Don't be scared of getting "too close" to people you love. CF

When it comes to sex-time things: if *you* don't want to do it, you really seriously don't have to do it. Your partner's feelings might be hurt a little bit because you said no, but ultimately they will trust and respect you more because you were honest about your preference and you shared your feelings with them. Anything less than an enthusiastic "yes" should be considered a "no thank you". And anyone who reacts poorly when you say "no thank you" is a person who does not respect your boundaries, and therefore does not need to be in your life. SS

You're not imagining it, allos really are just weird. Also being perceived in a sexual manner never gets any less inexplicable or off-putting, but at least now you don't have to put up with it in the expectation that it'll somehow morph into attraction on your part. DC

You don't need to rush. There is so much to learn and explore. It's okay to try labels and if you try something and you realize later on it doesn't fit you after all, that's okay. You are perfect as you are even if you have trouble describing what you are. You are perfect as you are even if you are unlike people around you and unlike what people expect of you. HBJ

Trust yourself, you really are ace. DE

Yes, you can also be bi at the same time. No, you don't have to like one girl for every boy to be a real bisexual. LG

It's okay to not come out. It's okay to never come out. You do not owe anyone an explanation and it's not your fault that they assume you're not queer. You are not any less queer by keeping it to yourself and staying safe. AB

I would [tell] her, or them, to be gentle with themselves. There is value in the knowing, when the knowing comes, but value in the learning, too. CD

Resources

Web-based resources

advocatesforyouth.org/wp-content/uploads/2019/03/ITIMB-ACE.pdf

azejournal.com

www.yasminbenoit.co.uk

autismserenity.tumblr.com

historicallyace.tumblr.com/about

www.campuspride.org/resources/introduction-to-asexual-identities-resource-guide

www.thetrevorproject.org/resources/article/understanding-asexuality

www.thetrevorproject.org/research-briefs/asexual-and-ace-spectrum-youth

Groups and organisations

www.asexuality.org AVEN, the Asexuality Visibility and Education Network

https://taaap.org The Ace and Aro Advocacy Project

https://acesandaros.org

www.asexuals.net An ace dating site
https://asexualoutreach.org Asexual Outreach
https://asexualgroups.wordpress.com (under construction)
www.meetup.com/topics/aromantic Aromantic meetups throughout the world
www.meetup.com/TGMAADM The Gay Men's Asexual and Demisexual Meetup
www.meetup.com/London-Asexuality-Meetup
www.meetup.com/Scotland-Asexual-Meetup

Nonfiction books and articles about a-spec identities

Andrews, A.K. (ed.) (2015) *Ace & Proud: An Asexual Anthology*. Purple Cake Press.

asexuals.net (n.d.) The history of asexuality. www.asexuals.net/the-history-of-asexuality

Bellamy, S. (2017) *Asexual Perspectives: 47 Asexual Stories*. Quirky Books.

Bogaert, A. (2021) *Understanding Asexuality*. Lanham, MD: Rowman and Littlefield.

Burgess, R. (2021) *How to Be Ace: A Memoir of Growing Up Asexual*. London: Jessica Kingsley Publishers.

Carrigan, M., Gupta, K. and Morrison, T.G. (2014) *Asexuality and Sexual Normativity: An Anthology*. Abingdon: Routledge.

Cerankowski, K.J and Milks, M. (eds) (2014) *Asexualities: A Queer and Feminist Perspective*. New York/Abingdon: Routledge.

Chen, A. (2021) *Ace: What Asexuality Reveals about Desire, Society, and the Meaning of Sex*. Boston, MA: Beacon Press.

Decker. J.S. (2015) *The Invisible Orientation*. New York, NY: Skyhorse Publishing.

Przybylo, E. (2019) *Asexual Erotics: Intimate Readings of Compulsory Sexuality*. Columbus, OH: University of Ohio Press.

Rothblum, E.D. and Brehony, K.A. (eds) (1993) *Boston Marriages: Romantic but Asexual Relationships Among Contemporary Lesbians*. Boston, MA: University of Massachusetts.

Scherrer, K.S. (2008) "Coming to an Asexual Identity: Negotiating Identity, Negotiating Desire." *Sexualities* 11, 5, 621–641. www.ncbi.nlm.nih.gov/pmc/articles/PMC2893352

Resources on sexuality more generally

Foucault, M. (1976/2020) *The History of Sexuality*: Volume 1: An Introduction. London: Penguin.

Foster, T.A. (2013) *Documenting Intimate Matters: Primary Sources for a History of Sexuality in America*. London: University of Chicago Press.

Institute of Historical Research, School of Advanced Study, University of London (n.d.) Catalogue: History of Sexuality and LGBTQ Collections. www.history.ac.uk/library/collections/sexuality

Seward, G.H. (1946) *Sex and the Social Order*. McGraw-Hill.

Weeks, J. (2016) *What is Sexual History?* Cambridge: Polity Press.

A-spec podcasts

A-OK

The Ace Couple

Sounds Fake but Okay

www.podchaser.com/lists/ace-rep-107ZzsCTjw – there's loads here, too many to cite!

A-spec YouTube channels

AmeliaAce
Aaron Ansuini
Chandler N Wilson
Christine Sydelko
Cody Daigle-Orians
Damian/HeyoDamo
Echo Gillette
Ellie Berry
Embly99
Evan Edinger
Lily and Saskia
Marshall John Blount
Nik Hampshire
Rowan Ellis
Samantha Aimee
Vesper/Queer as Cat

Fictional media that includes significant a-spec representation (though not necessarily a main character)

Radio Silence, Alice Oseman (book)
Loveless, Alice Oseman (book)
Bojack Horseman (TV series)
Sex Education (TV series)
Riverdale (comics, run from 2016, not TV series)
Summer Bird Blue, Akemi Dawn Bowman (book)
Elatsoe, Darcie Little Badger (book)
Not Your Backup, C.B. Lee (book, Sidekick Squad #3)

The Outer Worlds, Obsidian Entertainment (video game)
Every Heart a Doorway, Seanan McGuire (book)
Hazel's Theory of Evolution, Lisa Jenn Bigelow (book)
The Midnight Bargain, C.L. Polk (book)
The Tropic of Serpents, Marie Brennan (book)
She-Ra and the Princesses of Power (TV series)
Tash Hearts Tolstoy, Kathryn Ormsbee (book)
Let's Talk About Love, Claire Kann (book)
How to Be a Normal Person, TJ Klune (book)
Sirens (TV show)
The Movement, Gail Simone and Freddie Williams III (comics, DC)
Girls with Slingshots, Danielle Corsetto (book)
Common Bonds: A Speculative Aromantic Anthology, Claudie Arsenault, C.T. Callahan, B.R. Sanders and RoAnna Silver (editors) (book)
Rick, Alex Gino (book)
The Lady's Guide to Petticoats and Piracy, MacKenzie Lee (book)
The Birds, the Bees and You and Me, Olivia Hinebaugh (book)
The Adventure Zone: Graduation, the McElroy family (podcast)
March Family Letters (YouTube series)
Epithet Erased (YouTube series)
Steven Universe, Rebecca Sugar (TV series)
The Baker Thief, Claudie Arseneault (book)
Supernormal Step (webcomic series)
Tarnished Are the Stars, Rosiee Thor (book)
Hazbin Hotel (YouTube series)
The Art of Saving the World, Corinne Duyvis (book)
How to Say Goodbye in Robot, Natalie Standiford (may not be explicitly ace, but it is implied)
Bloom Into You (Yagate Kimi ni Naru), Nio Nakatani (manga and anime series)

Resources on coming out

www.youtube.com/watch?v=Kox1NMdBVgg
www.aromanticism.org/en/news-feed/coming-out-advice
https://thecoupleconnection.net/coming-out-as-asexual
https://whenicameout.com/tag/aromantic
www.asexualise.com/how-to-come-out-as-asexual
www.wikihow.com/Come-Out-As-Asexual-(for-Teenagers)

Resources on a-spec allyship

https://acesandaros.org/resources/a-beginner-s-guide-to-being-an-aromantic-ally
https://hr.qmul.ac.uk/media/hr/edi/Ace-Inclusion-and-Ally-ship-Booklet-.pdf
https://lgbtqia.ucdavis.edu/educated/ally-tips
https://nextstepcake.wordpress.com/2020/01/30/allyship-the-little-things-count-a-lot
www.aromanticism.org/en/printables
www.stonewall.org.uk/about-us/news/six-ways-be-ally-asexual-people

The following are a few more tips from my interviewees about how to help the a-spec people around you feel more safe and supported:

> Friends in particular should be really clear about what our relationship means to them because I often feel like I'm more invested in friendships than the other person. BH

> I think it's important to not compare different types of

relationships with one another and create a hierarchy of importance... I hate nothing more than to lose friends because they started to date and suddenly I became "unimportant" or "not a priority" because the relationship we had was "just" platonic. I care extremely deeply about my friends and these situations break my heart. AB

It feels so supportive when friends feel like they can make ace jokes with me, or mention it casually. Some of my friends (and honestly more so my family), while generally supportive, don't really feel like they can bring it up in conversation with me, or they get kind of uncomfortable if I bring it up. EL

My housemate once sent me a "happy ace day" text on the appropriate day, and that was nice – it makes you feel seen, you know? PQ

Be aware of what sex really is: it's not a need. It's not a pillar in a relationship. It's not a reason for every action of every person. It's just something we do because we want to. LL

They can stop pressur[ing] us [to] date someone or hook up with someone, and accept that not having sex does not make us immature or childish or pitiful. CF

Don't infantilise us. EF

Don't make it about you. HBJ

Don't make a big deal out of it. DE

Further reading on the relationship between the a-spec and LGBTQIA+ communities

https://historicallyace.tumblr.com
https://slate.com/human-interest/2020/03/asexuality-history-internet-identity-queer-archive.html
www.stonewall.org.uk/about-us/news/asexuality-queerest-thing

Further reading on sexual health for asexual people

Conley-Fonda, B. and Leisher, T. (2018) "Asexuality: sexual health does not require sex." *Sexual Addiction & Compulsivity* 25, 1, 6–11. DOI: 10.1080/10720162.2018.1475699
https://lgbt.foundation/sexualhealth
https://theeyeopener.com/2019/02/asexual-people-have-sexual-health-concerns-too

Further reading on a-spec identity, polyamory and relationship anarchy

http://theanarchistlibrary.org/library/andie-nordgren-the-short-instructional-manifesto-for-relationship-anarchy
www.arocalypse.com/topic/1229-relationship-anarchy
www.asexuality.org/en/topic/65092-relationship-anarchy
https://azejournal.com/article/2020/3/22/significant-others-aspec-polyamory-and-relationship-anarchy
www.taylorfrancis.com/chapters/edit/10.4324/ 9780203869802-23/asexual-relationships-asexuality-polyamory-kristin-scherrer

www.thecut.com/2018/10/what-does-relationship-anarchy-mean.html
www.theodysseyonline.com/how-to-practice-relationship-anarchy

Further reading on the relationship between asexuality and sexual violence

https://asexualsurvivors.org/get-help/other-resources
https://femmefrugality.com/wp-content/uploads/2016/10/Asexual-IPV-Brochure_MAY2016.pdf
https://www.huffingtonpost.co.uk/entry/asexual-discrimination_n_3380551
https://resourcesforacesurvivors.tumblr.com
www.victimservicecenter.org/asexuality-and-sexual-violence
www.womenslaw.org/about-abuse/abuse-specific-communities/lgbtqia-victims/forms-abuse/what-forms-abuse-are-unique-1

Further reading on BDSM/kink values and philosophy

https://fetlife.com/team
https://smartsexresource.com/topics/bdsm-kink
www.psychologytoday.com/gb/blog/sex-sexuality-and-romance/201901/what-is-kink

Further reading and resources on a-spec identity, culture and race

Eng, D. (2001) *Racial Castration: Managing Masculinity in Asian America*. Durham and London: Duke University Press.

Foster, A.B., Eklund, A., Brewster, M.E., Walker, A.D. and Candon, E. (2019) "Personal agency disavowed: identity construction in asexual women of color." *Psychology of Sexual Orientation and Gender Diversity* 6, 2, 127–137. https://doi.org/10.1037/sgd0000310

http://blackyouthproject.com/black-asexuals-are-not-unicorns-there-are-more-of-us-than-we-know

https://azejournal.com/asexuality-and-race

https://blavity.com/why-we-must-amplify-black-asexual-women-and-give-the-support-they-need

https://docs.google.com/document/d/1A7qvP4qvu0njLrMjl8tD68hqOiFZC9c10Wt6uXXBscE/edit#

https://mediadiversified.org/2014/05/03/whats-race-got-to-do-with-it-white-privilege-asexuality

https://taaap.org/2021/10/24/ace-week-21-bipoc-aces

https://zora.medium.com/on-being-black-female-and-asexual-30fbfb018ad4

www.qwearfashion.com/home/thisiswhatasexuallookslike-part-10-black-aces-edition

www.youtube.com/channel/UCNGdR787fwF7BxC5yMwIPEg

Further reading on a-spec identity and gender

https://elephantbirdaro.wixsite.com/aromanticsurveys/aromantic-gender-experiences

https://journals.sagepub.com/doi/10.1177/1363460718790890

https://journals.sagepub.com/doi/full/10.1177/1363460718790890

www.asexuality.org/en/topic/97074-aromantics-and-gender-identity

www.asexuality.org/en/topic/208503-gender-and-asexuality

www.researchgate.net/profile/Anthony-Bogaert/publication/8220138_Asexuality_Prevalence_and_Associated_Factors_in_a_National_Probability_Sample/links/5460c7fc0cf27487b4525dac/Asexuality-Prevalence-and-Associated-Factors-in-a-National-Probability-Sample.pdf

www.researchgate.net/publication/281444223_Masculine_Doubt_and_Sexual_Wonder_Asexually-Identified_Men_Talk_About_Their_Asexualities

www.thecut.com/2015/10/complex-linguistics-campus-queer-movement.html

Endnotes

Introduction

1 Chen, A. (2021) *Ace: What Asexuality Reveals about Desire, Society, and the Meaning of Sex*. Boston, MA: Beacon Press, p. 110, citing Diamond, L.M. (2003) "What does sexual orientation orient? A biobehavioral model distinguishing romantic love and sexual desire." *Psychological Review* 110, 1, 173–192.

2 Castro-Peraza, M.E., García-Acosta, J.M., Delgado, N., Perdomo-Hernández, A.M. *et al.* (2019) "Gender identity: the human right of depathologization." *International Journal of Environmental Research and Public Health* 16, 6, 978; Suess Schwend, A. (2020) "Trans health care from a depathologization and human rights perspective." *Public Health Reviews* 41, 1; Drescher, J. (2015) "Out of DSM: depathologizing homosexuality." *Behavioral Sciences* 5, 4, 565–575.

3 Note: The actual term "HSDD" was coined in 1977 by sex therapist Helen Singer Kaplan, and in 2013 with the updated DSM-V, the disorder was split into "male hypoactive sexual desire disorder" and "female sexual interest/arousal disorder". American Psychiatric Association (ed.) (2013) "Male Hypoactive Sexual Desire Disorder, 302.71 (F52.0)." *Diagnostic and Statistical Manual of Mental Disorders, Fifth Edition*. Washington, DC: American Psychiatric Publishing.

4 American Psychiatric Association (ed.) (2013) "Male Hypoactive Sexual Desire Disorder, 302.71 (F52.0)." *Diagnostic and Statistical Manual of Mental Disorders, Fifth Edition*. Washington, DC: American Psychiatric Publishing.

5 Jaiswal, J. (2019) "Whose responsibility is it to dismantle medical mistrust? Future directions for researchers and health care providers." *Journal of Behavioral Medicine* 45, 2, 188–196. doi:10.1080/08964289.2019.1630357;

Kennedy, B.R., Mathis, C.C. and Woods, A.K. (2007) "African Americans and their distrust of the health care system: healthcare for diverse populations." *Journal of Cultural Diversity* 14, 2, 56–60. PMID: 19175244.

6 Vaginismusandsexuality (2014, August 22) "Corrective therapy" for asexuals from medical professionals. Tumblr.com. Retrieved May 11, 2022, from https://vaginismusandsexuality.tumblr.com/post/95393272898/corrective-therapy-for-asexuals-from-medical; Asexuality Archive (2014, August 24) The Comment Section: I'm Not A Doctor, But I Play One On The Internet. Asexuality Archive. Retrieved May 11, 2022 from www.asexualityarchive.com/the-comment-section-im-not-a-doctor-but-i-play-one-on-the-internet/#HormoneCheck; Decker, J.S. (2014, September 18) I love the smell of asexual invalidation in the morning. Retrieved May 11, 2022, from https://swankivy.tumblr.com/post/97751199490/i-love-the-smell-of-asexual-invalidation-in-the; Drugs.com (2021, May 3) Flibanserin. Drugs.com. Retrieved March 20, 2022 from www.drugs.com/mtm/flibanserin.html

7 Brotto, L.A. (2009) "The DSM Diagnostic Criteria for Hypoactive Sexual Desire Disorder in Women." *Archives of Sexual Behavior* 39, 2, 221–239. doi.org/10.1007/s10508-009-9543-1

8 Meixel, A., Yanchar, E. and Fugh-Berman, A. (2015) "Hypoactive sexual desire disorder: inventing a disease to sell low libido." *Journal of Medical Ethics* 41, 859–862.

9 MacInnis, C.C. and Hodson, G. (2012) "Intergroup bias toward 'Group X': evidence of prejudice, dehumanization, avoidance, and discrimination against asexuals." *Group Processes & Intergroup Relations* 15, 6, 725–743. doi.org/10.1177/1368430212442419; DePaulo, B. (2020) "Biased against asexuals? Let me count the ways." *Psychology Today Blog*; Mosbergen, D. (2017) "Battling Asexual Discrimination, Sexual Violence and 'Corrective' Rape." *HuffPost UK*, 7 December.

10 Matthews, L. (2021) The Role of the Nuclear Family in Western Europe's Economic Development. Mises Institute, 17 May. Retrieved March 20, 2022, from https://mises.org/power-market/role-nuclear-family-western-europes-economic -development

11 Thompson, A.K. (2021) The Marxist Perspective on The Family. Revise-Sociology. Retrieved March 20, 2022, from https://revisesociology.com/2014/02/10/marxist-perspective-family

12 National Council on Family Relations (2021) Toward Dismantling Family Privilege and White Supremacy in Family Science. Retrieved March 20, 2022, from www.ncfr.org/events/ncfr-webinars/toward-dismantling-family-privilege-and-white-supremacy-family-science

Visibility

1 Klein, J. (2021) Asexuality: the ascent of the "invisible" sexual orientation. BBC Worklife. Retrieved March 20, 2022, from www.bbc.com/worklife/article/20210507-asexuality-the-ascent-of-the-invisible-sexual-orientation

2 Olusola, O. (2021) "Stay Weird You Only Live Once": Yasmin Benoit on Being Alternative and Asexual. *AZ Magazine*, 25 February. Retrieved March 20, 2022, from https://azmagazine.co.uk/yasmin-benoit-interview

3 AVEN (2021, August 16) Indigenous aces in North America. AVEN Livestreams. Retrieved March 20, 2022, from www.youtube.com/watch?v=ZxjjUiPYV9w&t=6s

4 Shilton, A.C. (2019) "The Importance of Running in Native American Culture." *Women's Running*, 25 February. Retrieved March 20, 2022, from www.womensrunning.com/culture/first-runners-native-american-women

5 Bangor Daily News (2021) "The Invisibility of Indigenous People Is Harmful to All Americans." *Bangor Daily News*, 30 April. Retrieved March 20, 2022, from https://bangordailynews.com/2021/04/30/opinion/opinion-contributor/the-invisibility-of-indigenous-people-is-harmful-to-all-americans; Moffatt, G.K. (2019) Voice of Experience: Invisible People, Part 1: Native Americans. *Counseling Today*, 18 March. Retrieved March 20, 2022, from https://ct.counseling.org/2019/03/voice-of-experience-invisible-people-part-1-native-americans

Who Are We?

1 Frawley (2021, December 14) The language of asexuality before AVEN. Nothing Radical. https://nothingradical.blog/2021/05/04/the-language-of-asexuality-before-aven

2 Waters, M. (2020) "Finding Asexuality in the Archives." *Slate Magazine* 6 March. Retrieved May 10, 2022, from https://slate.com/human-interest/2020/03/asexuality-history-internet-identity-queer-archive.html; lesbianherstorian (2018, July 3). Lisa Ben. Retrieved March 20, 2022, from https://lesbianherstorian.tumblr.com/post/175482819467/activists-at-barnard-college-providing-labels

3 Homoerotic-Ads (2020, July 16) Asexuality is not an "internet identity", a fad, or fake. Vintage Homoerotic Ads. Retrieved May 10, 2022,

from https://homoerotic-ads.tumblr.com/post/623757702993166336/asexuality-is-not-an-internet-identity-a-fad

4 LibGuides (2022) Asexuality: About. Westport Library. https://westportlibrary.libguides.com/asexuality

5 sonofzeal (2021, May 18) History of the term "Demisexual". Asexuality.Org. Retrieved March 20, 2022, from www.asexuality.org/en/topic/213551-history-of-the-term-demisexual

6 Chu, E. (2014) "Radical Identity Politics: Asexuality and Contemporary Articulations of Identity." In K.J. Cerankowski and M. Milks (eds) *Asexualities: Feminist and Queer Perspectives*. New York/Abingdon: Routledge, p.88.

7 Tobias, K. (2015) "No Sex, Please – I'm Asexual." *BUST*, 19 June. Retrieved May 10, 2022, from https://bust.com/sex/14324-no-sex-please-i-m-asexual.html

8 Chu, E. (2014) *ibid.*, p. 87.

9 Jankowski, L. (2018, February 23) Interview: Gadriel. Asexual Artists. Retrieved May 10, 2022, from https://asexualartists.wordpress.com/2018/02/23/interview-gadriel

10 Walmsley, C. (2016) The queers left behind: How LGBT assimilation is hurting our community's most vulnerable. *HuffPost*, 21 July. Retrieved May 10, 2022, from www.huffpost.com/entry/the-queers-left-behind-ho_b_7825158

11 Humbleoats, H. (2016, February 26) Gold-star ace. Asexual Representation. Retrieved May 10, 2022, from https://humbleoats.wordpress.com/2016/02/26/gold-star-ace/comment-page-1

12 Savage, D. (2017, September 13) Dan Savage: Girls and Women and Sex. *East Bay Express*. Retrieved May 10, 2022, from https://eastbayexpress.com/dan-savage-girls-and-women-and-sex-2-1

13 Note: Though only 10 per cent of the 2020 Ace Census respondents.

Microlabels

1 Asexual spectrum Aegosexual (n.d.) LGBTQIA+ Wiki Fandom. Retrieved May 10, 2022, from https://lgbtqia.fandom.com/wiki/Asexual_spectrum#Aegosexual

2 Whythefuckisyouromeo, A. (2014, December 6). Autochoris is a bit of a mouthful... Aromantic Spectrum Awareness Week. Retrieved May 10, 2022, from https://arospecawarenessweek.tumblr.com/post/104463164552/autochoris-is-a-bit-of-a-mouthful

3 Flannigan, A.M. (2017, August 29) Alterous attraction. Our Queer

Stories. Retrieved May 10, 2022, from https://ourqueerstories.com/alterous-attraction
4 Cupiosexual (n.d.) LGBTQIA+ Wiki. Retrieved July 15, 2022, from https://www.lgbtqia.wiki/wiki/Cupiosexual
5 Queerplatonic relationship (n.d.) LGBTQIA+ Wiki. Retrieved May 10, 2022, from https://lgbtqia.fandom.com/wiki/Queerplatonic_relationship
6 Kaz (2010, December 24) A/romanticism. Kaz's Scribblings. Retrieved May 10, 2022, from https://kaz.dreamwidth.org/238564.html

When Language Isn't Enough

1 Ma, A. (2011) "Celtic spirituality: the relationship between Christian and Pagan faiths." *Kannen Bright* 2, 72–77.
2 Cerankowski, K.J. and Milks, M. (eds) (2014) *Asexualities: Feminist and Queer Perspectives, 1st edn*. New York and Abingdon: Routledge.

Coming (and Being) Out

1 Olusola, O. (2021, 25 February) "Stay weird you only live once": Yasmin Benoit on being alternative and asexual. *AZ Magazine*. Retrieved March 20, 2022, from https://azmagazine.co.uk/yasmin-benoit-interview
2 See: Newsome, T. (2015, July 7) 5 tips for dealing with parents who don't accept your sexuality. Bustle. Retrieved May 10, 2022, from www.bustle.com/articles/95062-5-tips-for-dealing-with-parents-who-dont-accept-your-sexuality; Spunout (2021, June 23) What should I do if someone doesn't accept me for being LGBTI+? Spunout. Retrieved May 10, 2022, from https://spunout.ie/lgbti/lgbti-resources/someone-doesnt-accept-being-lgbt

A-spec and the LGBTQ+ Community

1 Note: I'm aware there are subtle differences in meaning and connotation between "LGBT+" and "queer". For the purposes of this chapter, I won't dig too deeply into the semantics here. I'll specify when I am not using the terms interchangeably, as in when my interviewees themselves

differentiate, for example BC: "Queers are a lot more accepting of ace folks than the run-of-the-mill LGBT folks."

2 Note: There are a number of scanned primary sources on Tumblr compiled by user autismserenity, and here https://edesiderata.crl.edu/resources/archives-human-sexuality-and-identity

3 Katz, J.N. (2019, June 1) Carl Schlegel: The first U.S. gay activist, 1906–1907. OutHistory: It's About Time. Retrieved May 10, 2022, from https://outhistory.org/exhibits/show/schlegel/contents

4 Waters, M. (2020) "Finding Asexuality in the Archives." *Slate Magazine*, 6 March. Retrieved May 10, 2022, from https://slate.com/human-interest/2020/03/asexuality-history-internet-identity-queer-archive.html

5 lesbianherstorian (2018, July 3) Lisa Ben. Retrieved March 20, 2022, from https://lesbianherstorian.tumblr.com/post/175482819467/activists-at-barnard-college-providing-labels

6 MacInnis, C.C. and Hodson, G. (2012) "Intergroup bias toward 'Group X': Evidence of prejudice, dehumanization, avoidance, and discrimination against asexuals." *Group Processes & Intergroup Relations* 15, 6, 725–743. doi.org/10.1177/1368430212442419

7 Scarlett, A.O. (2020, October 27) Asexuality is the queerest thing. Stonewall. Retrieved May 10, 2022, from www.stonewall.org.uk/about-us/news/asexuality-queerest-thing

8 The Limited Times (2021, May 14) Homosexual Paragraph 175: Karl Heinrich Ulrichs, Germany's first gay activist. News RND. Retrieved May 10, 2022, from https://newsrnd.com/news/2021-05-14-homosexual-paragraph-175--karl-heinrich-ulrichs--germany-s-first-gay-activist.Byk_5MndO.html; UK Parliament (n.d.) Regulating sex and sexuality: the 20th century. Retrieved May 10, 2022, from www.parliament.uk/about/living-heritage/transformingsociety/private-lives/relationships/overview/sexuality20thcentury

9 Purks, E. (2021, August 30) Being asexual and being sex-positive aren't mutually exclusive. Healthline. Retrieved May 10, 2022, from www.healthline.com/health/healthy-sex/asexual-sex-positivity#sex-positivity

10 Milks, M. (2014) Introduction. In K.J. Cerankowski and M. Milks (eds) *Asexualities: Feminist and Queer Perspectives, 1st edn*. New York and Abingdon: Routledge, p.5.

11 Cerankowski, K.J. (2014) Introduction. In K.J. Cerankowski and M. Milks (eds) *Asexualities: Feminist and Queer Perspectives, 1st edn*. New York and Abingdon: Routledge.

12 Bennett, J. (2014) "'Born this way': queer vernacular and the politics of origins." *Communication and Critical/Cultural Studies* 11, 211–230. doi.org/10.1080/14791420.2014.924153

Intersectionality

1 Paramo, M. (2017, March 16) The asexual community is predominately white. Why? Medium. Retrieved May 10, 2022, from https://medium.com/@Michael_Paramo/interrogating-the-whiteness-of-the-asexual-community-b5765a71f62b
2 Owen, I.H. (2014) "On the Racialization of Asexuality." In K.J. Cerankowski and M. Milks (eds) *Asexualities: Feminist and Queer Perspectives*. New York and Abingdon: Routledge.
3 The Ace and Aro Advocacy Project (2021, October 24) Ace Week 2021 – aces of ethnic and racial minorities. Retrieved May 10, 2022, from https://taaap.org/2021/10/24/ace-week-21-bipoc-aces
4 Chen, A. (2021) *Ace: What Asexuality Reveals about Desire, Society, and the Meaning of Sex*. Boston, MA: Beacon Press.
5 Miller, K. (2015, October 5) Consistent sexual sacrifice. CT Pastors. Retrieved May 10, 2022, from www.christianitytoday.com/pastors/2015/fall/consistent-sexual-sacrifice.html; Mother Teresa of Calcutta (n.d.) Priestly Celibacy: Sign of the Charity of Christ. Vatican. Retrieved March 20, 2022, from www.vatican.va/roman_curia/congregations/cclergy/documents/rc_con_cclergy_doc_01011993_sign_en.html
6 AVEN (2021, August 16) Indigenous aces in North America. AVEN Livestreams. Retrieved March 20, 2022, from www.youtube.com/watch?v=ZxjjUiPYV9w&t=6s
7 Butler, K. (2021, January 31) Being aroflux & Black. AUREA. Retrieved March 20, 2022, from www.aromanticism.org/en/news-feed/being-aroflux-and-black
8 Lloyd, C.M., Alvira-Hammond, M., Carlson, J. and Logan, D. (2021) Family, Economic, and Geographic Characteristics of Black Families with Children. *Child Trends*, 5 March. Retrieved May 9, 2022, from www.childtrends.org/publications/family-economic-and-geographic-characteristics-of-black-families-with-children
9 AVEN (2021, August 16) Indigenous aces in North America. AVEN Livestreams. Retrieved March 20, 2022, from www.youtube.com/watch?v=ZxjjUiPYV9w&t=6s
10 I use the word "racialisation" here to acknowledge that what we are taught

to call "race" is a social construct. The concept of race was invented during the Industrial Revolution and the expansion of colonialism, during which new ideas about science and human beings as belonging to biological "types", with white people on top and people of colour below, were used to justify colonial violence. For more information see Roediger, D.R. (n.d.) Historical Foundations of Race. National Museum of African American History and Culture. Retrieved May 9, 2022, from https://nmaahc.si.edu/learn/talking-about-race/topics/historical-foundations-race

11 Kivel, P. (2017) *Uprooting Racism: How White People Can Work for Racial Justice, 4th edn*. Gabriola Island, BC: New Society Publishers.

12 Owen, I.H. (2014) "On the Racialization of Asexuality." In K.J. Cerankowski and M. Milks (eds) *Asexualities*. New York and Abingdon: Routledge.

13 See for example: Blackburn Center (2019, February 5) Girlhood interrupted: On R. Kelly and how Black girls are viewed in our society. Retrieved May 9, 2022, from www.blackburncenter.org/post/2019/02/05/girlhood-interrupted-on-r-kelly-and-how-black-girls-are-viewed-in-our-society; Epstein, R., Blake, J. and Gonzalez, T. (2017) "Girlhood interrupted: the erasure of Black girls childhood." *SSRN Electronic Journal*. doi.org/10.2139/ssrn.3000695; Blake, J.J. and Epstein, R. (2019) *Listening to Black Women and Girls: Lived Experiences of Adultification Bias*. Initiative on Gender Justice & Opportunity. Retrieved May 9, 2022, from www.law.georgetown.edu/poverty-inequality-center/wp-content/uploads/sites/14/2019/05/Listening-to-Black-Women-and-Girls.pdf

14 Kee, J. (1998) "(Re)sexualizing the desexualized Asian male in the works of Ken Chu and Michael Joo." *Jouvert*. Retrieved May 9, 2022, from https://legacy.chass.ncsu.edu/jouvert/v2i1/KEE.HTM

15 US NARA (2022, February 17) Chinese Exclusion Act (1882). National Archives. Retrieved May 9, 2022, from www.archives.gov/milestone-documents/chinese-exclusion-act

16 The Take (n.d.) The "Asexual" Asian Man – end the undesirable stereotype. Retrieved May 9, 2022, from https://the-take.com/watch/the-asexual-asian-man-end-the-undesirable-stereotype

17 Vaid-Menon, A. (2018, November 19) What's r(ace) got to do with it? white privilege & (a)sexuality. Media Diversified. Retrieved May 9, 2022, from https://mediadiversified.org/2014/05/03/whats-race-got-to-do-with-it-white-privilege-asexuality

18 Note: This essay is speaking specifically to the experiences of Asian men, but Vaid-Menon themself is gender-nonconforming and transfeminine.

19 Chen, A. (2021) *Ace: What Asexuality Reveals about Desire, Society, and the Meaning of Sex*. Boston, MA: Beacon Press, p.71.

20 Including one person who wrote "Man or male, 2001 Honda Civic DX" – I'm not sure if it was a joke, but it made me laugh.

21 Wilson, B.D.M. and Meyer, I.H. (2021, June 1) Nonbinary LGBTQ adults in the United States. Williams Institute. Retrieved May 9, 2022, from https://williamsinstitute.law.ucla.edu/publications/nonbinary-lgbtq-adults-us

22 Gender Minorities Aotearoa (2021, August 29) [Mis]Representation of transgender women in films. Retrieved May 9, 2022, from https://genderminorities.com/2017/04/03/misrepresentation-of-transgender-women-in-films; Walters, M.A., Paterson, J., Brown, R. and McDonnell, L. (2020) "Hate crimes against trans people: assessing emotions, behaviors, and attitudes toward criminal justice agencies." *Journal of Interpersonal Violence* 35, 21–22, 4583–4613. doi:10.1177/0886260517715026; FeelPrettyOnThursday (2022, January 22) Struggling with feeling sexualised. Reddit. Retrieved May 9, 2022, from www.reddit.com/r/MtF/comments/saeou5/struggling_with_feeling_sexualised; Crossdreamers, referencing Laube *et al.* (2020) "Sexual behavior, desire, and psychosexual experience in gynephilic and androphilic trans women: a cross-sectional multicenter study." *Journal of Sexual Medicine* 17. 10.1016/j.jsxm.2020.01.030

23 Nico-Nico Friendo, L. (2007, July 3) Biological Sex Poll (July 2007) Asexual Visibility and Education Network. Retrieved May 9, 2022, from www.asexuality.org/en/topic/24599-biological-sex-poll-july-2007; Bianchi, T. (2018) "Gender Discrepancy in Asexual Identity: The Effect of Hegemonic Gender Norms on Asexual Identification". WWU Honors Program Senior Projects. 81. Retrieved May 9, 2022, from https://cedar.wwu.edu/wwu_honors/81

24 Harper, A. and Proctor, C. (2012) *Medieval Sexuality: A Casebook.* New York and Abingdon: Routledge; Karras, M.R. (2017) *Sexuality in Medieval Europe: Doing unto Others, 3rd edn.* New York and Abingdon: Routledge.

25 Decameron Web Society (2011, January 31) Sexual desire. Retrieved May 9, 2022, from www.brown.edu/Departments/Italian_Studies/dweb/society/sex/sexual-desire.php

26 Kranzberg, M. and Hannan, M.T. (n.d.) History of the organization of work – women in the workforce. Encyclopedia Britannica. Retrieved March 26, 2022, from www.britannica.com/topic/history-of-work-organization-648000/Women-in-the-workforce; Burnette, J. (2008, March 26) Women workers in the British Industrial Revolution. EH.Net Encyclopedia, edited by Robert Whaples. Retrieved May 9, 2022, from http://eh.net/encyclopedia/women-workers-in-the-british-industrial-revolution

27 Women and industrialisation (n.d.) Warwick Department of History. Retrieved May 9, 2022, from https://warwick.ac.uk/fac/arts/history/students/modules/hi253/lectures/lecture2

28 Note: This is a simplification of the gender dynamics of the Industrial Revolution – race and class also had a huge role in shaping the lived experience of both men and women during this time.

29 Furneaux, H. (2014, May 15) Victorian sexualities. The British Library. Retrieved March 26, 2022, from www.bl.uk/romantics-and-victorians/articles/victorian-sexualities; Studd, J. and Schwenkhagen, A. (2009) "The historical response to female sexuality." *Maturitas* 63, 2, 107–111. Retrieved May 9, 2022, from doi.org/10.1016/j.maturitas.2009.02.015; FGRLS CLUB (2019, April 17) It's not us, it's history: Women's sexuality through the years. Retrieved May 9, 2022, from https://fgrlsclub.com/2019/04/its-not-us-its-history-womens-sexuality-through-the-years

30 Koedt, A. (1970) Myth of the Vaginal Orgasm. CWLU HERSTORY. Retrieved May 9, 2022, from www.cwluherstory.org/classic-feminist-writings-articles/myth-of-the-vaginal-orgasm

31 Kühl, S. (n.d.) *The Angel in the House and Fallen Women: Assigning Women their Places in Victorian Society.* [ebook] pp.171–178. Retrieved May 9, 2022, from https://open.conted.ox.ac.uk/resources/documents/angel-house-and-fallen-women-assigning-women-their-places-victorian-society

32 Note: Generally, the only women I've encountered in listicles about "asexual historical figures" are Florence Nightingale, Emily Brontë, Emma Trosse and possibly Queen Elizabeth I.

33 Click (n.d.) Changing Sexual Attitudes and Options. Retrieved May 9, 2022, from www.cliohistory.org/click/body-health/sexual?video=1862&cHash=f04bb12d0e378503749b0f24aaad1069

34 Broster, A. (2021) What Is the Orgasm Gap? Forbes, 10 December. Retrieved May 10, 2022, from www.forbes.com/sites/alicebroster/2020/07/31/what-is-the-orgasm-gap; SBS Australia (2012) Women Seen as Sex Objects: Scientific Studies. SBS News, March 26. Retrieved September 8, 2022, from www.sbs.com.au/news/article/women-seen-as-sex-objects-scientific-studies/848tbfmwv; Prendergast, C. (2021) What Is the Orgasm Gap? Here's How Sexual-Tech Is Making Pleasure More Inclusive. *British Vogue*, February 16. Retrieved May 10, 2022, from www.vogue.co.uk/beauty/article/the-orgasm-gap

35 Showden, C.R. (2016) "Feminist Sex Wars." In A. Wong, M. Wickramasinghe, r. hoogland and N.A. Naples (eds) *The Wiley Blackwell Encyclopedia of Gender and Sexuality Studies.* doi.org/10.1002/9781118663219.wbegss434

36 p.53.

37 Przybylo, E. (2014) "Masculine Doubt and Sexual Wonder: Asexually-Identified Men Talk About Their (A)sexualities." In K.J. Cerankowski and M. Milks (eds) *Asexualities: Feminist and Queer Perspectives.* New York and Abingdon: Routledge, p.231.

38 Lang, C. (2018) Intimacy and Desire Through the Lens of an Aro-Ace Woman of Color. Honors Theses. 252. Retrieved May 10, 2022, from https://scarab.bates.edu/honorstheses/252; Fisher, G. (2021) "I Felt There Was Something Wrong With Me": What It's Like to Be Aromantic but Not Asexual. *Metro*, February 26. Retrieved May 10, 2022, from https://metro.co.uk/2021/02/26/what-its-like-to-be-aromantic-its-different-from-being-asexual-14145314; Borresen, K. (2021) What It Means to Be "Aromantic," According to Aromantic People. *HuffPost UK*, June 16. Retrieved May 10, 2022, from www.huffingtonpost.co.uk/entry/what-does-it-mean-to-be-aromantic_n_5bb501cee4b01470d04de20d

39 Przybylo, E. (2014) "Masculine Doubt and Sexual Wonder: Asexually-Identified Men Talk About Their (A)sexualities." In K.J. Cerankowski and M. Milks (eds) *Asexualities: Feminist and Queer Perspectives*. New York and Abingdon: Routledge.

40 In Henriques, J., Hollway, W., Venn, C. and Walkerdine, V. (1984) *Changing the Subject*. London: Methuen. Via Przybylo.

41 Przybylo, E. (2014) "Masculine Doubt and Sexual Wonder: Asexually-Identified Men Talk About Their (A)sexualities." In K.J. Cerankowski and M. Milks (eds) *Asexualities: Feminist and Queer Perspectives*. New York and Abingdon: Routledge, p.236.

42 Przybylo, E. (2014) *ibid.*, p.232.

43 Przybylo, E. (2014) *ibid.*, p.233.

44 Sodha, S. (2021) Romantic Partner? Who Needs One When It's Friends Who Truly Help Us Get Through Life. *The Guardian*, 24 October. Retrieved May 10, 2022, from www.theguardian.com/commentisfree/2021/oct/24/romantic-partner-who-needs-one-when-its-friends-who-truly-help-us-get-through-life

45 Mayer, D. (2018) How Men Get Penalized for Straying from Masculine Norms. *Harvard Business Review*, 9 October. Retrieved May 10, 2022, from https://hbr.org/2018/10/how-men-get-penalized-for-straying-from-masculine-norms; McCreary, D.R. (1994) "The male role and avoiding femininity." *Sex Roles* 31, 517–531. doi.org/10.1007/BF01544277

46 Note: I'm mindful that this is a simplification of the role of men – of course race and socioeconomic status among others play a part in who gets to be seen as masculine and who gets to be seen as a sexual agent.

47 Siggy (2013, December 9) Oh the stars that you can earn! The Asexual Agenda. Retrieved May 10, 2022, from https://asexualagenda.wordpress.com/2013/12/09/oh-the-stars-that-you-can-earn

48 Alessa-lemur (2020, March 20) Pride Month!! Alessa is asexual? by alessa-lemur. Furaffinity. Retrieved May 10, 2022, from www.furaffinity.net/view/32023982; WellThisWentWell, W.T.W.W. (2021, January 4) If your child

came out as an asexual, how would you feel/react? Mumsnet. Retrieved May 10, 2022, from www.mumsnet.com/Talk/am_i_being_unreasonable/4022363-If-your-child-came-out-as-an-asexual-how-would-you-feel-react?pg=9; Why do so many think asexual is an actual sexual orientation, when it's technically a term to describe a form of sexual impotence? Why is... (2021, March 20) Quora. Retrieved May 10, 2022, from www.quora.com/Why-do-so-many-think-asexual-is-an-actual-sexual-orientation-when-it-s-technically-a-term-to-describe-a-form-of-sexual-impotence-Why-is-it-a-part-of-the-LGBTQ-spectrum

49 Lane, C. (2021, October 27) Why I'm founding Disabled Ace Day. Ace Week. Retrieved May 10, 2022, from https://aceweek.org/stories/why-i-m-founding-disabled-ace-day

50 Brook (2019) Young people with a learning disability are being denied sex-positive RSE. Brook, 12 September. Retrieved May 10, 2022, from https://legacy.brook.org.uk/press-releases/young-people-with-a-learning-disability-are-being-denied-sex-positive-rse; Campbell, M., Löfgren-Mårtenson, C. and Martino, A.S. (2020) "Cripping sex education." *Sex Education* 20, 4, 361–365. doi.org/10.1080/14681811.2020.1749470; Addlakha, R., Price, J. and Heidari, S. (2017) "Disability and sexuality: claiming sexual and reproductive rights." *Reproductive Health Matters* 25, 50, 4–9. doi.org/10.1080/09688080.2017.1336375; Rowlands, S. and Amy, J.J. (2017) "Sterilization of those with intellectual disability: evolution from non-consensual interventions to strict safeguards." *Journal of Intellectual Disabilities* 23, 2, 233–249. doi.org/10.1177/1744629517747162; Brady, S.M. (2001) "Sterilization of girls and women with intellectual disabilities." *Violence Against Women* 7, 4, 432–461. doi.org/10.1177/10778010122182541

51 Henriques-Gomes, L. (2020) "We Are Sexual Beings": Why Disability Advocates Want the NDIS to Cover Sexual Services. *The Guardian*, 21 April. Retrieved May 10, 2022, from www.theguardian.com/australia-news/2019/jul/22/we-are-sexual-beings-why-disability-advocates-want-the-ndis-to-cover-sexual-services; Samuel, M. (2021) Care staff helping disabled people access sex work services not breaking law, rules court. *Community Care*, 5 May. Retrieved May 10, 2022, from www.communitycare.co.uk/2021/05/05/care-staff-helping-disabled-people-access-sex-work-services-breaking-law-rules-court

52 See: Barounis, C. (2014) "Compulsory Sexuality and Asexual/Crip Resistance." In K.J. Cerankowski and M. Milks (eds) *Asexualities: Feminist and Queer Perspectives, 1st edn.* New York and Abingdon: Routledge; Kim, E. (2014) "Asexualities and Disabilities in Constructing Sexual Normalcy," *ibid.*; Gupta, K. (2014) "Asexuality and Disability: Mutual Negation in *Adams v. Rice* and New Directions for Coalition Building," *ibid.*

53 Disabled World (2021, December 23) Autism: neurodiversity and pathology paradigms. Retrieved May 10, 2022, from www.disabled-world.com/health/neurology/autism/paradigms.php

54 Rusting, R. (2021) Decoding the overlap between autism and ADHD. Spectrum Autism Research News, 2 August. Retrieved May 10, 2022, from www.spectrumnews.org/features/deep-dive/decoding-overlap-autism-adhd; Leitner, Y. (2014) "The co-occurrence of autism and attention deficit hyperactivity disorder in children – what do we know?" *Frontiers in Human Neuroscience 8*. doi.org/10.3389/fnhum.2014.00268

55 McAlpine, M.K. (2018, December 17) Autistic ≠ asexual. Medium. Retrieved May 10, 2022, from https://marykatemcalpine.medium.com/autistic-asexual-3a9488435b2a; Brilhante, A.V.M., Filgueira, L.M.D.A., Lopes, S.V.M.U. *et al.* (2021) "'Eu não sou um anjo azul': a sexualidade na perspectiva de adolescentes autistas." ("'I am not a blue angel': sexuality from the perspective of autistic adolescents.") *Ciência & Saúde Coletiva (Science Health Collect)* 26, 2, 417–423. doi.org/10.1590/1413-81232021262.40792020

56 Attanasio, M., Masedu, F., Quattrini, F., Pino, M.C. *et al.* (2021) "Are autism spectrum disorder and asexuality connected?" *Archives of Sexual Behavior*. doi.org/10.1007/s10508-021-02177-4; George, R. and Stokes, M.A. (2017) "Gender identity and sexual orientation in autism spectrum disorder." *Autism* 22, (8), 970–982. doi.org/10.1177/1362361317714587

Friends and Family

1 IrrationalPoint, via Kaz (2010, December 24) A/romanticism. Kaz's Scribblings. https://kaz.dreamwidth.org/238564.html

2 Note: I like this way of describing the relationship hierarchy not only because of IrrationalPoint's clear and unapologetic language but also because their description recalls the tone of religious dogma, which I find very fitting.

What Is Love?

1 No. 2: Gezelligheid (n.d.) Stuff Dutch People Like. Retrieved March 25, 2022, from https://stuffdutchpeoplelike.com/2015/09/23/gezelligheid-gezellig

2 Amae Psychology Wiki Fandom (n.d.) Psychology Wiki. Retrieved March 25, 2022, from https://psychology.fandom.com/wiki/Amae

3 Rotter, J. (2021, September 12) Ciğerpare. Departures. Retrieved May 10, 2022, from www.departures.com/travel/cigerpare

4 BBC Culture (n.d.) The "untranslatable" Japanese phrase that predicts love. Retrieved March 25, 2022, from www.bbc.com/culture/article/20180103-the-untranslatable-japanese-phrase-that-predicts-love

5 Babylangues (2019, April 15) Untranslatable – la douleur exquise. Retrieved March 25, 2022, from https://job-in-france.babylangues.com/intraduisibles/untranslatable-la-douleur-exquise; The Bucharest Lounge (2015, February 28) The meaning of the Romanian word "Dor", according to four Transylvanian women. Retrieved March 25, 2022, from https://bucharestlounge.wordpress.com/2015/02/28/the-meaning-of-the-romanian-word-dor-according-to-four-transylvanian-women

6 Brueckner, A. (2014) 13 Untranslatable Words That Have to Do With Love. Thought Catalog, 17 February. https://thoughtcatalog.com/alex-brueckner/2014/02/13-untranslatable-words-that-have-to-do-with-love

7 The Intrepid Guide (2020, August 14) 203 most beautiful untranslatable words [the ultimate list: A–Z]. Retrieved May 10, 2022, from. www.theintrepidguide.com/untranslatable-words-ultimate-list

8 Neos Kosmos (2017) The eight types of love according to the ancient Greeks. Neos Kosmos, February 3. Retrieved May 10, 2022, from https://neoskosmos.com/en/2017/02/03/news/greece/the-eight-types-of-love-according-to-the-ancient-greeks%20; Krznaric, R. (2022) Love Like a Greek: The Six Types of Love. *GreekReporter*, 20 January. Retrieved May 10, 2022, from https://greekreporter.com/2022/01/20/six-types-love-ancient-greece

9 Hirji, S. and Krishnamurthy, M. (2021) What Is Romantic Friendship? *New Statesman*, 22 November. Retrieved May 10, 2022, from www.newstatesman.com/ideas/agora/2021/11/what-is-romantic-friendship

10 Murdoch (1968), via Hirji and Krishnamurthy, *ibid.*

11 Theophano, T. (2004) Boston Marriages. glbtq. Retrieved May 10, 2022, from www.glbtqarchive.com/ssh/boston_marriages_S.pdf

12 Jenkins, C. (2017) *What Love Is: And What It Could Be*, 1st edn. New York: Basic Books.

13 Hirji and Krishnamurthy, *ibid.*, paraphrasing Jenkins.

14 Historicallyace (2021, April 18) What Kind of Attraction? A History of The Split Attraction Model. Aceing History. Retrieved May 10, 2022, from https://historicallyace.tumblr.com/post/648763527373504512/what-kind-of-attraction-a-history-of-the-split

15 Note: This confusion can actually extend to sexual attraction as well. HD, who is demiromantic ace, says, "I kind of thought sexual attraction was something people were lying or joking about throughout middle school.

I had never felt it and thought people around me were making things up to sound cool/more mature. I would lie to fit in when people asked me which boys I thought were 'hot' or 'sexy'."

16 Chu, E. (2014) "Radical Identity Politics: Asexuality and Contemporary Articulations of Identity." In K.J. Cerankowski and M. Milks (eds) *Asexualities: Feminist and Queer Perspectives*. New York and Abingdon: Routledge.

17 Chu, E. (2014) *ibid.*, page 90.

18 www.lgbtqia.wiki/wiki/Alterous_Attraction

19 www.lgbtqia.wiki/wiki/Quoiromantic

Sex

1 Older Than Netfic (2021, May 17) Some thoughts on asexuality, kink, and queer inclusion. Retrieved May 10, 2022, from https://olderthannetfic.tumblr.com/post/651362946032746497/some-thoughts-on-asexuality-kink-and-queer; Jolene Sloan, L. (2015) "Ace of (BDSM) clubs: building asexual relationships through BDSM practice." *Sexualities 18*, 5–6, 548–563. doi.org/10.1177/1363460714550907; Brunning, L. and McKeever, N. (2020) "Asexuality." *Journal of Applied Philosophy 38*, 3, 497–517. doi.org/10.1111/japp.12472

2 Note: For more information, see this *Independent* article advocating against kink at pride (notably written by a known TERF): Baker-Jordan, S. (2021) BDSM and Kink Don't Belong in Pride Celebrations. This Is Why. *The Independent*, 25 May. Retrieved May 10, 2022, from www.independent.co.uk/voices/bdsm-kink-pride-lgbt-rights-celebrations-why-b1853859.html, as well as a queer-perspective analysis from Insider and Vox Haasch, P. and López, C. (2021) The Debate Over "Kink at Pride" Divides the Internet, but the Kink Community Has Been Part of Queer Protest and Celebration Since Stonewall. *Insider*, 7 June. Retrieved May 10, 2022, from www.insider.com/kink-at-pride-discourse-explained-kinks-role-in-lgbtq-history-2021-6; Abad-Santos, A. (2021) The Perpetual "Kink at Pride" Discourse, Explained. *Vox*, 2 June. Retrieved May 10, 2022, from www.vox.com/the-goods/22463879/kink-at-pride-discourse-lgbtq

3 Mosbergen, D. (2013) Battling Asexual Discrimination, Sexual Violence And "Corrective" Rape. *Huffington Post*, 20 June; Doan-Minh, S. (2019) Corrective Rape: An Extreme Manifestation of Discrimination and the State's Complicity in Sexual Violence, 30 Hastings Women's L.J. 167. Retrieved May 10, 2022, from https://repository.uchastings.edu/hwlj/vol30/iss1/8; Galop (2021) Acephobia and anti-asexual hate crime. Retrieved May 10, 2022, from https://galop.org.uk/resource/acephobia-and-anti-asexual-hate-crime

4 Hille, J.J., Simmons, M.K. and Sanders, S.A. (2020) "'Sex' and the ace spectrum: definitions of sex, behavioral histories, and future interest for individuals who identify as asexual, graysexual, or demisexual." *The Journal of Sex Research* 57, 7, 813–823, DOI: 10.1080/00224499.2019.1689378

5 Barker, M.J. (2019, November 15). Asexuality and trauma – Meg-John and Justin. Meg-John & Justin. Retrieved May 10, 2022, from https://megjohnandjustin.com/you/asexuality-and-trauma; Flannigan, A.M. (2017, August 29) Misconceptions & stereotypes surrounding asexuality. Our Queer Stories. Retrieved May 10, 2022, from https://ourqueerstories.com/misconceptions-stereotypes-surrounding-asexuality; Script LLGBTT (2018, March 21) FAQ – What are the stereotypes of asexual and aromantic characters? Retrieved May 10, 2022, from https://scriptlgbt.tumblr.com/post/172084355431/faq-what-are-the-stereotypes-of-asexual-and; and in media, for example the film *Mysterious Skin*: www.imdb.com/title/tt0370986

6 Australian Human Rights Commission (2017) Change the Course: National Report on Sexual Assault and Sexual Harassment at Australian Universities 2017. Australian Human Rights Commission.

7 Sangya Project (2021, August 25) Asexuality and kink. Retrieved May 10, 2022, from www.sangyaproject.com/home/asexuality-kink; AceofHeartss (2016, March 10) Asexual BDSM. Asexual Visibility and Education Network. Retrieved May 10, 2022, from www.asexuality.org/en/topic/134841-asexual-bdsm; Kaden (2007, November 24) Asexual BDSM & kink. Asexual Visibility and Education Network. Retrieved May 10, 2022, from www.asexuality.org/en/topic/27065-asexual-bdsm-kink

The Future of Relationships

1 Kaz (2010, December 24) A/romanticism. Kaz's Scribblings. Retrieved May 10, 2022, from https://kaz.dreamwidth.org/238564.html

2 Smith, S.E. (2021, September 14) I don't mean to baffle you, but I do: queerplatonic partnerships. This Ain't Livin'. Retrieved May 10, 2022, from http://meloukhia.net/2012/06/i_dont_mean_to_baffle_you_but_i_do_queerplatonic_partnerships

3 Ndabane, T. (2021) I'm Single, But I Get All the Romance I Need From My Friendships. *Refinery29*, 10 August. Retrieved May 10, 2022, from www.refinery29.com/en-gb/2021/08/10621575/romantic-friendships-platonic-love; Sodha, S. (2021) Romantic Partner? Who Needs One When It's Friends Who Truly Help Us Get Through Life. *The Guardian*, 24 October. Retrieved May 10, 2022, from www.theguardian.com/commentisfree/2021/oct/24/romantic-partner-who-needs-one-when-its-friends-who-truly-help-us-get-through-life; Hirji, S. and Krishnamurthy, M. (2021) What Is Romantic Friendship? *New Statesman*, 28 December. Retrieved May 10, 2022, from www.newstatesman.com/ideas/agora/2021/11/what-is-romantic-friendship

4 Ross-Barrett, J. (2020, April 16) Significant others: Aspec, polyamory and relationship anarchy. AZE. Retrieved May 10, 2022, from https://azejournal.com/article/2020/3/22/significant-others-aspec-polyamory-and-relationship-anarchy

5 Note: The form of polyamory discussed in this chapter is specifically non-hierarchical polyamory, which assumes equal importance to each individual relationship.

6 See Sidhu, P. (2020, September 22) 10 books about polyamorous and open relationships. Electric Literature. Retrieved May 10, 2022, from https://electricliterature.com/10-books-about-polyamorous-and-open-relationships/; Persaud, I. (2020) Top 10 Novels about Unconventional Families. *The Guardian*, 15 April. Retrieved May 10, 2022, from www.theguardian.com/books/2020/apr/15/top-10-novels-about-unconventional-families; Vishwathika (2018, May 15) These 8 films with unconventional families are a delight to watch. Get Started with These...Women's Web: For Women Who Do. Retrieved May 10, 2022, from www.womensweb.in/2018/05/what-does-it-take-to-make-a-family

7 Nordgren, A. (2012, August 14) The short instructional manifesto for relationship anarchy. The Anarchist Library. Retrieved May 12, 2022, from http://theanarchistlibrary.org/library/andie-nordgren-the-short-instructional-manifesto-for-relationship-anarchy

Joy

1 Benoit, Y. (2021) #ThisIsWhatAsexualLooksLike Part 10: Black Aces Edition. Qwear Fashion, 14 November. Retrieved May 12, 2022, from www.qwearfashion.com/home/thisiswhatasexuallookslike-part-10-black-aces-edition

2 Aces&Aros (2018, October 27) Asexual Awareness Week, day six. Retrieved May 12, 2022, from https://aces-and-aros.tumblr.com/post/179460713784/asexual-awareness-week-day-six-most-of-these-are

3 Ohana, R. (1998) Golden Orchid Society. Rainbow Rumpus [online] 8. Retrieved May 12, 2022, from www.rainbowrumpus.org/html/political09.htm; Wolf, A.P., Martin, E. and Ahern, E.M. (1978) *Studies in Chinese Society*. California: Stanford University Press.

Index